Cultural Issues in Healthcare

Renay Scales • Asia T. McCleary-Gaddy
Editors

Cultural Issues in Healthcare

Emerging Challenges and Opportunities

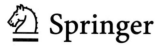 Springer

Editors
Renay Scales, PhD
(Formerly UK-COM)
Associate Professor of Family and
Community Medicine
Plano, TX, USA

Asia T. McCleary-Gaddy, PhD
Office of Diversity and Inclusion
UT McGovern School of Medicine
Houston, TX, USA

ISBN 978-3-031-20825-6   ISBN 978-3-031-20826-3   (eBook)
https://doi.org/10.1007/978-3-031-20826-3

This Springer imprint is published by the registered company Springer Nature Switzerland AG
The registered company address is: Gewerbestrasse 11, 6330 Cham, Switzerland

Preface

The motivation for this publication began in 2012 when the opportunity to redesign and teach a community and behavioral medicine course as part of clinical course offerings at an Undergraduate Medical Education (UME) institution. The research that ensued to determine the gaps in what was recently part of the curriculum led to disparaging results. Very little about health disparities for marginalized and underserved populations was being provided to medical students, who if successful in their matriculation, would be degreed doctors. Existing resources used for clinical medicine courses braised the surface of rituals and traditions related to births and deaths that healthcare providers had come to know about treating patients with diverse religious practices. One of the largest bodies of examination in this regard addressed dietary practices including those that were part of faith celebrations, surgical practices or prohibitions, and end-of-life rituals that attending medical personnel needed to be aware of. Metropolitan Chicago Healthcare Council summarized these practices by faith categories as part of an advisory to providers.

After being selected as a national clinical faculty in family medicine by the National Board of Osteopathic Medical Examiners (NBOME) in 2013 and beginning to write and review national board exam questions about ethical policy, practice, and procedure, it was clear that interest existed for more curricular inclusion of this material so that students and residents could be better prepared to address disparities by understanding population health issues and concerns. This new energy from national medical leaders including those at NBOME further supported a need for new [text] books to resource students and faculty in all medical education programs while the American Hospital Association and other healthcare delivery organizations calling for standards inclusive of these communication and ethical practices. Increased venues for interprofessional education further made the case for studying-related issues. Currently, a national online medical education program is providing significant study materials to address diversity, equity, and inclusion for UME students. This material includes definitions, examples of how these issues impact health and healthcare providers, and specific provisions to aid in addressing disparities.

Outreach to prospective authors to submit chapters on topics within their special areas of expertise that would align with the vision for a supplemental textbook for professional healthcare education and training programs. These chapters will address current and emerging cultural issues in medicine and will add to the body of knowledge on population health and care.

Plano, TX, USA   Renay Scales
Houston, TX, USA   Asia T. McCleary-Gaddy

Acknowledgments

We are indebted to the women and Dr. Dexter James, who entrusted their research and scholarship with us over the last 3 years. When the pandemic hit, it slowed many elements of progress in the country, and the world, and even completely halted projects like ours. We had to figure out how to continue teaching and learning in a completely virtual environment, adjust to working from home while at the same time addressing the altered needs of our families and ourselves, and all of this mostly in isolation. How do medical, dental, nursing, pharmacy and other health-care students, trainees, residents, and interns get the on-the-job, hands-on training that they need, in the midst of an environment where exposure to COVID 19 and its variants could mean their very lives—our lives. It required a great deal of ingenuity and patience.

Renay Scales

My gratitude is extended to all the medical students, interprofessional education (pharmacy, nursing, social work, optometry, and medica) students in my sessions, doctoral students, and residents that I have taught or trained for all that I learned in relationship with them, and all clinical and science faculty that allowed me to infuse cultural consciousness into their work. It was these experiences that afforded me a national clinical faculty nomination by Dr. William Betz and acceptance by the National Board of Osteopathic Medicine Examiners (NBOME), and the incredible opportunity to write and review board questions for level 1, 2, and 3. I am thankful for their support in assessing students and residents through competence in cultural aspects of behavioral and ethical practices that increase efficacy with patient populations that have been underserved.

As this book was being visioned, Dr. Roberto Cardarelli, my *Family and Community Medicine* Chair at the University of Kentucky College of Medicine, and Dr. Karen Roper, colleague respectively afforded me the assigned time to conduct the calls to potential contributors and the many documents that had to be prepared to ensure that chapters answered the questions that connected to the purpose of the book as well as assistance with early edits. Karen struggled with me through guiding the first five authors through edits that better connected their work to the book's vision.

I have profound appreciation for each of the 13 authors, several of which, started with me over 3 years ago. If the pandemic was not enough of a challenge, they waited through a year of catastrophic illnesses that disabled me from moving the book forward. They could have decided, of course, to take their work to another venue. It was particularly tough on those in aggressive promotion and tenure environments to hang in with me.

As I encountered the opportunity to meet, co-author, and support Asia in her research and career, I noticed the incredible potential she possessed as a resource and partner. I asked her to join this last year. Her energy, enthusiasm, and ability brought the needed rebirth of the project. I have heartfelt gratitude for her willingness to join in as co-editor.

Lastly, but in no way least, I always give honor to God, my family, and to my faithful community for cheering me on in all endeavors in my life.

Asia T. McCleary-Gaddy

I would like to acknowledge my fiancé Ronald Bright II for supporting me through this venture and encouraging me to "think big." I would also like to thank my mother, Letricia McCleary for her continuous prayers over my mind, body, and spirt. I love you both! I would also like to thank Renay for inviting me to the book as co-editor, and to the incredible scholars that I have interacted with in our progress.

Contents

Editors and Contributors

About the Editors

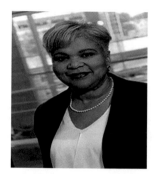 **Renay Scales, Ph.D.** has served on three (3) presidential teams and in other leadership capacity in corporate, healthcare, and higher education organizations. Her leadership responsibilities have included talent acquisition and management relations, faculty relations, and development and DEI. She has also taught or trained undergraduate, graduate, and doctoral students and medical students and residents on organizational and practice behavior, leadership, and health equity-related competencies. She named a national clinical faculty member in family medicine by the National Board of Osteopathic Medical Examiners (NBOME); she writes and reviews all levels of board exam questions in ethics and jurisprudence. Scales had oversight of a global health program between a former U.S. initiative and the University of KwaZulu Natal in South Africa.Dr. Scales' work has been acknowledged through a best practice award by OCR, MLK Civil Leadership Awards, a Barrier Breaker Award, and recently, was acknowledged by the National Accrediting Commission for Diversity and Inclusion as Professional of the Month during Women's History Month. She is a former member of the National Advisory Council for the National Conference on Race and Ethnicity (NCORE) and former board member of the National Coalition Building Institute (NCBI). Her role as a leadership consultant includes work with more than 70 organizations. Scales' research and scholarship

primarily addresses health equity with a focus on cultural traumas. She has widely presented her research and practice and was recently the keynote for the International Association of Medical and Science Education's annual conference.

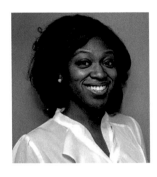

Asia T. McCleary-Gaddy, Ph.D. serves as the Director of Diversity and Inclusion for UTHealth and Assistant Professor of Psychiatry and Behavioral Sciences for McGovern Medical School. Asia serves the UTHealth community through design and implementation of policies and procedures that support diversity and inclusion, recruitment, and retention of URM faculty and students, program evaluation, and data analysis for students, residents, and faculty members. Dedicated to furthering the empirical research published on diversity and health, she has published in leading journals including Annals of Behavioral Medicine, Journal of Health Psychology, and Equality, Diversity, and Inclusion.Previously, Dr. McCleary-Gaddy served as the inaugural Director of Diversity and Equity for Hackensack Meridian School of Medicine and helped launch the institution's high school pipeline/pathway programs. Prior to that role, she served as a Data Analyst for the Vermont Department of Health in Burlington, VT where she analyzed data for the Healthy People 2020 initiative. Dr. McCleary-Gaddy earned a PhD in Experimental Social Psychology. She also holds a Bachelor of Arts in Psychology with a distinction in Research and Creative Works from Rice University.

Contributors

Michelle Douglas Human Resources and EDI, Florida State University, Tallahassee, FL, USA

B. DaNine J. Fleming The Medical University of South Carolina, Diversity, Equity and Inclusion, Charleston, SC, USA

Idella G. Glenn Equity and Inclusion—Office of the President, University of Southern Maine, Portland, ME, USA

Monica D. Griffin Charles Center, William and Mary, Williamsburg, VA, USA

Lisa M. Hooper Center for Educational Transformation, University of Northern Iowa, Cedar Falls, IA, USA

Drexler James Assistant Professor of Psychology, Univeristy of Minnesota, Twin Cities, Minneapolis, MN, USA

V. Faye Jones Department of Pediatrics, University of Louisville School of Medicine, Louisville, KY, USA

Katie F. Leslie Sullivan University College of Pharmacy and Health Sciences, Louisville, KY, USA

Asia T. McCleary-Gaddy Psychiatry and Behavioral Sciences, McGovern Medical School at the University of Texas Health Science Center at Houston, Houston, TX, USA

Diversity and Inclusion, McGovern Medical School at the University of Texas Health Science Center, Houston, TX, USA

Rebecca Oliver-Lemieux OB/GYN, TriHealth, Cincinnati, OH, USA

Paige Rentz Center for Leadership and Social Change, Florida State University, Tallahassee, FL, USA

Renay Scales University of Kentucky College of Medicine (Formerly), Lexington, KY, USA

University of North Texas Health Science Center, Contractor for Leadership Development Coaching, Plano, TX, USA

Ava Stanzak Primary Care, Kansas College of Osteopathic Medicine, Wichita, KS, USA

Tukea L. Talbert Office of Executive VP for Health Affairs, University of Kentucky HealthCare, Lexington, KY, USA

Chapter 1
Introduction

Renay Scales

Background

After addressing an overarching issue of race trauma and its physiological manifestations as a result of cumulative micro and macro aggressions [1], it became noticeable how we fail to regard these issues with clients and patients in the healthcare arena. Patriarchal systems often refute these phenomena or relegate them to creations of individual imagination. Some health providers began to acknowledge the potential benefit of a deeper examination of the impact of trauma from racism, classism, sexism, and homophobia on already vulnerable and challenged patient populations. Moving to another academic medical college and providing training for physicians, scientists, and residents, an even more stark realization of the absence of curriculum on cultural consciousness in healthcare or key information about healthcare disparities further ignited a desire to resource healthcare educators, students, trainees and acting physicians and other healthcare professionals with these data. As this book proceeded to review by our publisher, the change in the title from "medicine" to "healthcare" came from the understanding that these topics were needed in the education and training of all health professionals. For example, these data are helpful in training public health practitioners, social workers, nurses, pharmacists, optometrists, medical students and residents, and others who make up medical treatment teams.

The purpose of this book is to examine emerging cultural issues in healthcare for marginalized patient populations. We explore the impact of community and family beliefs on healthcare decisions and outcomes, provide further knowledge on social determinants of health, and report some best practices in community medicine. The authors are currently in practice as physicians, behaviorists, researchers, and other

R. Scales (✉)
University of North Texas Health Science Center, Contractor for Leadership Development Coaching, Plano, TX, USA

professionals who are infusing cultural competency into healthcare principles and practice. They are physicians, nurses, psychologists, behavioral medicine practitioners, and other leaders in the subject matter explored in this publication within various institutions or private practice within the United States.

As we reviewed other books that address cultural issues in healthcare, we only found two other resources that we located that address as diverse topics in the field as this book. We seek to include information on issues that are even more current than those in other publications.Additional resources for those developing current-day strategies for patient care will be helpful in improving the quality of care for all patients.

Why is Culture Important in Health and Healthcare?

Historical Treatment

When the social determinants of health are considered, particularly those that relate to community factors such as income, education and other quality of life indicators reported by the CDC, it is clear that cultural beliefs and behaviors of patient populations are important in achieving positive health outcomes [2]. Health and disease are addressed, however, unequally historically in the United States. Proactive wellness and early interventions needed to reduce disease is less accessible by racialized, low socioeconomic or poor people. Such inequity has fueled health disparities for some patient communities. These gaps in the healthcare status and/or outcomes for these and other groups as a result of the historical lack of access to preventative and overall quality patient care [3].

One such example relates to women. Historically, not only have the doctors, scientists, and researchers been male, but most of the human and animal cell studies have been from male species, making data released [inappropriately] generalized to female biology [4]. This adds to the problematic nature of health for women. Even with the specialization of maternal health, vestiges of misinformation exist today. Affluence in society is also allowing a widening gap to develop between the health of the white and nonwhite populations [5].

Using members of vulnerable populations in the United States for dangerous testing is also part of the history of treatment related to healthcare. The Tuskegee Experiment covering a 40-year time span used black men without their knowledge, to determine an effective treatment for syphilis. Not only were they never told the truth about the study, but treatment known to be effective was withheld from participants.

In another example of historical mistreatment, Henrietta Lacks' cells were regenerated and sold for sizable amounts of money, without her consent. Later, her descendants suffered their own illnesses without the affordability of healthcare. Other examples exist involving the mistreatment of children and military personnel who were looking to prolong their deployment to war zones. They agreed to participate in studies on agents of biomedical warfare without being fully informed of the potential danger to their health. Homeless people, refugees, and other poor people were similarly used for research without being told about the process and possible detrimental outcomes [6].

Cultural and Gender Bias

Even though medical professionals make vows and take oaths to provide respectful treatment to all patients, bias and stereotypes play a part in their delivery of healthcare [7]. From emergency care to obstetrics and pain management, biases have a detrimental impact on how doctors treat people of color [4]. The same is true another report states, for treatment by male providers to women patients. A staffer at The Guardian, Gabrielle Jackson [8], writes about how male bias in medical trials ruined women's health. She references the book, Doing Harm, by Maya Dusenbery. The publication demonstrates how bad science and medicine have discounted women through misinformation and dismissal of [their] reports of sickness. It further states that male professionals insert "hysteria" into their considerations for physical illness of female patients.

The culture of marginalized groups is a much bigger indicator than we once believed when it comes to behavior related to healthcare. Culture is learned behavior shared with group members across generations [9]. Similarly, culture is defined by Hernandez and Gibb [10] as a socially transmitted system of shared knowledge, beliefs, and/or practices that vary across groups which have been a significant factor in adapting for, in our case, humans across the history of our existence. What is believed about the industry of medicine, the providers, and treatment measures as well as what providers' biases are regarding patient populations impact access, perceived quality of care and trust in providers, and how providers treat patients. Given these factors, to provide culturally competent care requires providers and healthcare organizations to deliver services that meet the belief-based, social, and other related needs of patients and their families to increase the quality of outcomes [11]. How to build effective relationships between healthcare providers and patients is one of the greatest challenges of modern medicine given that the country is becoming more and more diverse in language, culture, and the practice of traditions related to their distinct ancestries [12].

Student and Workforce Diversity

Having more diverse students and trainees in the health professions is a motivation to examine the impact of one's culture on health and healthcare. In a large-scale international study on motivation for seeking medical education, among the top reasons were those relating to the students' families and communities [13]. Those seeking medicine and other health professions, evidenced in many of the personal statements in their applications, are moved by personal experiences. Some have had their own encounters with healthcare challenges, others have witnessed or even engaged those of their families and friends in a way that motivated their careers. While economic resource is also a goal according to one study, cultural reasons are a rising theme behind interest in these fields. For example, recent data reported of the absence of healthcare professionals of color and from rural areas. Recruitment efforts for healthcare programs, consequently, are focusing on outreach to these communities for education and training that will increase their participation in these professions [14]. Medical, dental, optometry, nursing, and other healthcare professional schools benefit by having an increase in the trained healthcare workforce and patients benefit by having a more diverse pool of healthcare providers.

Impact of Cultural Diversity on Patients

One model addresses the relationship between diversity of providers and how patients feel about care [15]. Nguyen reports that an increased sense of cultural consciousness extending from diverse learners, trainees, and providers enables a greater sense of safety among patients, especially when they have linguistic and cultural differences from the more dominant provider group identities. One such example is awareness of Appalachian culture among healthcare providers.

An examination of Appalachian history and healthcare is an example of how patient concerns arise when feelings of distrust are a barrier to healthcare-seeking behavior. People indigenous to this vast region of the U.S. have a diversity that is unaddressed by many other sources that write about cultural aspects of the region. Ways of living and behaving, are better understood when we have accurate information about the history and traditions of the group(s) [16]. While socioeconomic class impacts all people who have less than enough financial resources to get and understand quality affordable care, there are places in Appalachia that still lack access to healthcare. This lack of access coupled with beliefs and other less than positive ways of thinking about healthcare have caused areas within this region to carry some of the most significant, life-threatening comorbidities in the country. Even when people who have grown up under these practices are better able to acquire quality care, negative feelings about health-seeking can continue to serve to increase the causes of disease and other debilitating conditions.

Erin Prather [17], in her cover story for Texas Medical Association's publication, describes an Asian woman who utilized a mammography mobile unit from the University of Texas M.D. Anderson Cancer Center learned she had a concerning film of her breast that needed to be explained to her so that she would agree to more tests. The patient was upset, thinking she had contracted breast cancer while on the van. The article goes on to make an important point that there are rarely if ever "bad" patients. There are, however, misunderstood ones who require understanding from their providers and better communication to enable successful outcomes. One word, and occasionally shift in tone, can change the meaning of an expression in many languages.

In Damon Tweedy's book, *Black Man in a White Coat...* [18] he shares some of the lived experiences he encounters in the process of obtaining his medical education and training in medical school and as a resident and fellow. He speaks early in the book about lingering after class, one he had been in for months, to engage his professor. The professor assumed he was there to repair an item in the classroom. He continues to further chronicle the many micro and macroaggressions he encounters. Cumulatively, these aggressive acts can create such despair that one, as did Tweety, can begin to wonder if they are good enough or worthy of such accomplishments [1].

As the casual reader or trainee utilizing this material as a supplement required by a healthcare education program encounters reports of disparity among the various chapters, the hope is that examples and stories may also create empathy for the conditions in which people are vulnerable to being discounted or otherwise engaged in a less than thoughtful or respectful manner in their pursuit of health, and how they are made to feel frustrated and distrustful of providers. Even the providers who represent these groups find themselves distrusting of colleagues on their teams.

"Of course, these residents are idiots, they've been trained by a woman," one male surgeon says about his female colleague in the operating room in the presence of a team of medical staff.

An example of how, in this case, a woman surgeon is subjugated at work. A ripple effect for other female personnel present also occurred in this instance. Thankfully, the patient was not yet conscious. Nonetheless, the practitioner and trainees were slammed publicly.

The "Me Too" movement and "Time is Up," spotlighted in 2019, was only the tip of the iceberg in what happens in medicine across gender lines. The jokes, memes, and other behavior that emanates from a lack of cultural consciousness are harmful to colleagues, patients, and even patient families if they are in earshot of the comments [19].

This is our attempt to avert these behaviors and replace them with ones that represent the empathy so many professions seek to have resonated among certified, licensed healthcare professionals providing direct patient care.

Culturally Responsive Teaching and Training

Teaching and training with the outcome of increased cultural competency can be challenging.

Muniz [20] names needed competencies: (1) Reflect on one's cultural lens, (2) Recognize and redress bias in the system, (3) Draw on students' culture to share curriculum and instruction, (4) Bring real-world [healthcare] issues into the classroom, (5) Model high expectations for all students, (6) Promote respect for students' differences, (7) Collaborate with families and the local community, and (8) Communicate in linguistically and culturally responsive ways. While these are basic competencies suggested across varying levels and types of education, they can be found in the models of community medicine spotlighted in this book.

Chapters address the stigma that often extends from a lack of understanding or embedded stereotypes, which adversely affects marginalized, underserved, or otherwise vulnerable populations. Presented here are women, weight-oppressed individuals, LGBT plus communities, mentally challenged patients, Black and Hispanic/LatinX, youth and other identities. Becoming even more aware of these disparities will clarify the need for increased knowledge and competence engaging these communities. Outcomes can improve, we believe, with cultural consciousness. Effectively communicating with and treating these community members is a critical consideration in the training and education of all healthcare professionals.

Chapters are comprised of historical data, nominal reports of aggregated data, best practice models, and clinical anecdotes, and are rooted in qualitative and evidence-based research. The content addresses healthcare communication in provider–patient relationship, mental health, healthcare management, and comfort care, as well as the more general aspects of bias that impact collegial and patient encounters. The subtext is derived from the collective direct experiences of the authors, barring interviewers of those directing model programs. Refer to the appendices for short bios of the authors.

Summary of the Contents

For the ease of distinguishing subject matter in coordination with your syllabus, chapters can be organized into the following subcategories:

Historical Nature of a Single Vulnerable Community and the Impact on Health Outcomes

Adolescent Mental Health and Culturally Responsive Pediatric Care
> Treatment of Women in Healthcare Environments.
> The Commoditization of Blacks and the Impact on Health Outcomes.

Characteristics of Care: Anecdotal and Scholarly Strategies for Training Professionals

Appalachian Care.
> A Culture of Stigmatization: The Healthcare of Minoritized Populations.
> Transgender Healthcare: Can We Achieve High-Performing Healthcare Delivery to All?

Cultural Models that Address Quality of Care

Brown Bodies in Pain and the Call for Narrative Medicine.
> Models of Community Care.

References

1. Davis, M., Vakalahi, V., & Scales, R. (2015). Women of color in the academy: from trauma to transformation. In K. De Welde & A. Stepnick (Eds.), *Disrupting the culture of silence: Confronting gender inequality and making change in higher education* (pp. 265–277). Stylus.
2. USA.gov, last reviewed September 2021. CDC Social determinants of health: know what affect health.
3. Riley, W. (2012). Health disparities: Gaps in access, quality, and affordability of medical care. *Transactions of the American Clinical and Climatological Association, 123*, 167–172.
4. Rees M. Racism in healthcare: What you need to know. Medical News Today. 2020.
5. Cornely, P. (2011). The health status of the negro today and in the future. *American Journal of Public Health, 101*(S1), 161–163.
6. Pence, G. E. (2010). *Medical ethics: Accounts of groundbreaking cases* (Vol. 10, 6th ed., pp. 177–185). McGraw-Hill.
7. Chapman, E., Katz, A., & Carnes, M. (2013). Physicians and implicit bias. *Journal of General Internal Medicine, 28*(11), 1504–1510.
8. Jackson, G. (2019). The female problem: How male bias in medical trials ruined women's health. *The Guardian*, 13.
9. Berlinger, N., & Berlinger, A. (2017). Culture and moral distress: What's the connection and why does it matter? *AMA Journal of Ethics, 19*(6), 608–616. Medicine and Society.
10. Hernandez, M., & Gibb, J. (2019). Culture, behavior and health. *Evolution, Medicine, and Public Health, 2020*(1), 12. Oxford Academic.
11. Swihart, D. L., Yarrarapu, S. N. S., & Martin, R. L. (2021). *Cultural religious competence in clinical practice* (p. 2). StatPearls Publishing.
12. Johnson, T. (2019). *The importance of physician-patient relationships, communication and trust in health care*. Duke Center for Personalized Care (posted on Mach 11).
13. Goel, S., Angeli, F., & Ruwaard, D. (2018). What motivates medical students to select medical studies: A systematic literature review. *BMC Medical Education, 18*, 16.
14. Stowers, T., Lyndon, M., Henning, M., Hill, A., & Webber, M. (2019). Exploring factors that motivate and influence medical students to attend medical school. *The Asian Pacific Scholar, 4*(3), 3–12.
15. Nguyen, H. (2008). Patient centered care-cultural safety in indigenous health. *Australian Family Physician, 37*(12), 990–994.
16. McGarvey, E., Leon-Verdin, M., Killos, L., Guterbock, T., & Cohn, W. (2011). Health disparities between Appalachian and non-Appalachian counties in Virginia USA. *Journal of Community Health*. pubmed.ncbi.nlm.nih.gov › 20862529, *36*(3), 348–356. https://doi.org/10.1007/s10900-010-9315-9
17. Prather, E. (2006). Keep your guard up. *Texas Medical Association, 102*(4), 45–46. PMID: 17128757.
18. Tweedy, D. (2015). *Black man in a white coat: A doctor's reflection on race and medicine*. Picador.
19. Gupta, R., Gupta, A., & Nehra, D. (2019). Going forward with the #me too movement: Toward a safer work environment. *Journal of Psychosexual Health, 1*(2), 174–179.
20. Muñiz, J. (2019). *Culturally responsive teaching: a 50-state survey of teaching standards*. newamerica.org/education-policy/reports/culturally-responsive-teaching/2: https://www.newamerica.org/creative-commons/.

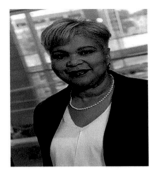

Dr. Renay Scales has served on three (3) presidential teams and in other leadership roles, and as faculty for many years. She has had responsibility for faculty development/faculty affairs (including at universities with unionized faculty); as Division Chief for Talent Management and Diversity, Equity and Inclusion; and as a faculty member teaching organizational behavior, leadership, and health equity related courses for medical students and residents, masters, and doctoral students.

Dr. Scales has also served as faculty and as a dean in a medical college, teaching culturally responsive patient care to medical students and training residents on population health, and was administratively responsible for the development of physicians and scientists for over a decade. She was named a national clinical faculty member in family medicine with NBOME where she writes and reviews board exam questions for all levels of board exams. Scales has worked in academic medicine, business and industry, and all genres of higher education. A global health program addressing the prevention and treatment of HIV/AIDS in partnership with the University of KwaZulu Natal in South Africa is among her proudest accomplishments.

Dr. Scales' work has been acknowledged through a *Best Practice* award by OCR, MLK Civil Leadership Award, a *Certificate of Excellence* from American Society for Bioethics and Humanities, and recent acknowledgements from the National Accrediting Commission for Diversity and Inclusion as Professional of the Month during Women's History Month. She is a former member of the National Advisory Council for the National Conference on Race and Ethnicity (NCORE) and former board member of the National Coalition Building Institute (NCBI). In the role as a leadership consultant to C suite professionals includes more than 80 academic, clinical, and other organizations. Scales' research and scholarship focuses primarily on bias and stigma with recent articles and book chapters on race trauma and mental health. She has widely presented her research and practice and was recently the keynote for the International Association of Medical and Science Education's annual conference.

Part I
Historical Nature of a Single Vulnerable Community and the Impact on Health Outcomes

Chapter 2
Adolescent Mental Health and Culturally Responsive Pediatric Care

V. Faye Jones, Katie F. Leslie, and Lisa M. Hooper ⓘ

Introduction

According to 2021 US Census Bureau estimates, there were approximately over 43,000,000 youth aged 10–19 in the United States, accounting for more than 13% of the total US population [1]. The growing diversity in racial and ethnic groups in the nation has been more pronounced in the child population than in the adult population with this trend projected to continue through 2060 [2]. It had been estimated that when the 2020 Census was conducted, more than half of the nation's children would be part of a minority race or ethnic group. What is even more striking is the projection by 2060 estimates that just 36% of all children under the age of 18 will be single-race non-Hispanic White, compared with 52% today [1, 2]. Consequently, there is an urgent need to infuse culture (e.g., language, race, and religion) into health assessment, prevention, intervention, and treatment models. Providers and others in the healthcare field must be aware of the demographic and cultural identities represented in the patient and community population (e.g., low-resourced, rural, bilingual, and severe poverty) they serve.

V. F. Jones
Department of Pediatrics, University of Louisville School of Medicine, Louisville, KY, USA
e-mail: Vfjone01@louisville.edu

K. F. Leslie
Sullivan University College of Pharmacy and Health Sciences, Louisville, KY, USA
e-mail: KLeslie@sullivan.edu

L. M. Hooper (✉)
Center for Educational Transformation, University of Northern Iowa, Cedar Falls, IA, USA
e-mail: lisa.hooper@uni.edu

R. Scales, A. T. McCleary-Gaddy (eds.), *Cultural Issues in Healthcare*,
https://doi.org/10.1007/978-3-031-20826-3_2

Toward this end, and contrary to previous trends in population expansion, a significant amount of this growth occurs outside the typical urban core counties of metropolitan areas [3]. Additionally, the percentage of adolescents living in low-income families has increased to 40% in 2014 compared to 35% in 2008, with 19% living below the poverty line [4]. Racial minority populations are affected more than majority populations with 60% of Black adolescents and 59% of Hispanic adolescents living in low-incomes families, with 33% of Black youth and 28% of Hispanic youth identified as living in poor families. This compares with only 27% of White adolescents living in low-income families, with 11% living in poor families [4]. In addition, 52% of adolescents of immigrant parents compared to 36% of adolescents of native-born parents live in low-income families [4]. These factors and others contribute to the continually changing patient profile about which providers and others in the healthcare field must have the knowledge, skills, and competencies that underpin culturally responsive pediatric care. The changing demographics in the United States will continue to have a major impact on the delivery of healthcare and public health initiatives. As the population continues to diversify, the nation will continue to see the impact on mental and medical health disparities and its effect on the families and communities being served.

As previously mentioned, the adolescent population is an important demographic on which this chapter focuses. In addition, given the unique developmental needs of adolescents, we consider the extent to which this life stage places adolescents in a particular vulnerable state as they experience physical changes, emotional stress, and ecological and contextual experiences (family, school, and community). The adolescent health literature suggests these factors are additive and intersect and thus they all ought to be considered in how mental health issues emerge and thus are assessed, diagnosed, and treated (see [5]). Providers and others in the healthcare field must be prepared to use ecologically valid interventions and culturally tailor other interventions (i.e., evidence-based) that appear to be efficacious and effective with White, middle-class youth but have yet to be tested and evaluated with racial and ethnic minority populations [6–8]. Health disparities have long existed but *may* be ameliorated or reduced if cultural adaptations are considered in pediatric mental health care [9].

Adolescence is described as a transitional stage between childhood and adulthood. It marks a time of significant physical and psychological changes, as well as cognitive growth. Adolescence is shaped by three phases of development: early, middle, and late adolescence. Changes are variable from individual to individual but usually begin and end around the second decade of life. Genetics, gender, race, and ethnicity contribute to and intersect with the timing of puberty but other factors, such as nutritional and environmental exposures from lived experiences impact development as well. All societies recognize this progression; however, the manner in which it is defined, acknowledged, and in some cases celebrated differs among cultural groups and societal expectations [10].

Biological Implications of Adolescence

The biological changes that are evidenced in adolescence are important. Typically, when one thinks of adolescence it is the physical changes that are seen; however, hormonal changes need to occur prior to the emergence of these observable physical changes. The function of the hypothalamus and the adrenal glands in hormonal regulation are critical for the physical expressions of puberty to be observed and referred to as gonadarche and adrenarche, respectively [11]. The hypothalamic-pituitary-gonadal axis controlling the hypothalamus gonadostat regulation is hypersensitive to low-dose sex steroid (androgens and estrogens) in childhood resulting in gonadotropin-releasing hormone (GnRH) suppression. This feedback loop prevents the release of luteinizing hormone (LH) and follicle-stimulating hormone (FSH). At the end of childhood, there is a change in the feedback sensitivity resulting in an escalation of GnRH. As the GnRH level surges, the pituitary gland increases the release of LH and FSH. As a consequence of their rise in concentration, sex steroids surge, either testosterone or estradiol, depending on the gender of the adolescent resulting in the physical changes of puberty. In males, LH promotes testosterone production. Sperm maturation occurs secondary to an increase in FSH. In females, an increase in both LH and FSH is needed for the ovaries to produce estrogen, progesterone, and small amounts of testosterone [11].

Although independent of the hypothalamic-pituitary-gonadal axis, the adrenal gland also increases the production of the adrenal androgens of dehydroepiandrosterone (DHA), dehydroepiandrosterone-sulfate (DHEA-S), and androstenedione [12]. These hormones are responsible for adult body odor, development of axillary and pubic hair, increased testicular size, and early changes in body growth [11, 12]. Hormonal activity occurs prior to the observable physical changes [11, 12]. Other hormones that play a role in puberty development include thyroid hormone, cortisol, glucagon, growth hormone and somatomedins and leptin [13, 14].

Developmental Implications of Adolescence

Equally important during adolescence are the psychosocial and cognitive developmental aspects that are observed. Developmental theorists have attempted to explain the psychosocial and cognitive development evidenced in adolescents [15–18]. The three stages of adolescent development—early, middle, and late—incorporate aspects of these theories to underscore the process the majority of adolescents experience on their pathway to adulthood. The following discussion considers the main features of these stages. However, it should be understood a distinct separation of the stages is not possible. Instead, there is frequent overlap and moving in and out of these phases throughout the progression to maturity and adulthood.

Early adolescence begins at approximately 10 years of age and ends around 13 years of age (i.e., the middle school years). This stage is underscored by the beginning of the physical and biological changes that were discussed earlier. The adolescent is concerned about self. They care about acceptance and belonging. Borrowing from the work of Barrett [19], this stage can be summarized in the question, "Am I normal?" Adolescents begin more complex processing, going from concrete thinking to more abstract thinking, although they are more focused on self and the present. During this stage, a moral compass is beginning to emerge with questions and challenges toward authority figures [19]. The adolescent may engage in limit testing, which may lead to experimentation with drugs and alcohol or other risky behaviors [20].

The hallmark of *middle adolescence* is the development of one's identity [19]. The adolescent is able to understand him/herself separate from others and discovers or clarifies: "What makes him/her unique?" [19]. The adolescent's self-esteem may be connected to their ability to recognize their own strengths and talents and may alternate between having high expectations for themselves compared to a feeling of failure in endeavors setting up an internal conflict [20]. Body image may be a primary focus coupled with a concern about appearance, including sexual attractiveness [20]. Conflicts with parents may increase with the adolescent placing lower importance on parents while elevating the importance of peer groups [20]. Additionally, during this period, abstract thinking predominates, which enhances the adolescent's ability to think about the meaning of life and set goals [19]. Intellectual interests tend to increase, which may set up inner conflicts related to academic abilities and performance [20]. In middle adolescence, the focus continues to be on self. The completion of physical development typically occurs during the next stage, late adolescence [21].

Late adolescence, the period of late high school/college, involves individuals planning for the future beyond their immediate environment. Adolescents are able to use abstract reasoning as they reflect on their own ideas and experiences. They have the capacity to appreciate humor, to make decisions independent of others and to compromise on issues [19, 20]. Also, this stage is marked by an ability to delay gratification. Late adolescence also is a stage where the adolescent may develop a feeling of worthiness because they are capable of living up to a moral code of right and wrong and proficient in the acceptance of social and cultural norms. Changes in this stage include heightened self-esteem, sexual maturity, planning for the future, and how to affect change [19, 20].

The intersection of biological and developmental states and identities taken together creates vulnerabilities for mental health conditions. As stated previously, adolescence is a period of significant changes resulting in the brain establishing more complex neural pathways and behavioral patterns that will last into adulthood [22]. It also is a time of increased stress associated with these changes and the adolescent attempting to navigate the expected developmental tasks creating an environment of increased risk for mental health concerns [23]. A confounding factor is the role of culture and how it intersects with biological and developmental states. Relevant cultural factors, which may be the adolescence's, their family, or both, and the adolescent's self-reported cultural identities may be implicated in how the adolescent copes with and reacts to stress. The interaction of culture can often support the well-being of the adolescent or inhibit coping to everyday and culturally relevant stressors, which places the adolescent at risk for the development of mental health disorders [23].

Cultural Implications of Adolescence

While a number of factors influence the development, diagnosis, and management of adolescent mental health disorders in the general population, certain population groups face additional mental health issues and healthcare disparities. A study by Lu reported higher rates of depression for females and older adolescents [24]. Additionally, research has shown that racial and ethnic minority adolescents are less likely to be diagnosed, seek out, and/or use mental health services [24–26]. The next section considers several vulnerable racial, ethnic, and cultural minority populations.

Socioeconomic Status

A social factor, such as family income, is a significant predictor of mental health status in children and adolescents [27–29]. In 2015, 20% of all children under 18 years of age were living in poverty defined as annual income of $24,300 for a family of four [30, 31] with 19% of adolescents ages 12 through 17 years living in poor families [4]. Forty-two percent of all children were living in low-income families, defined as 200% or less of the poverty threshold. This compares to 40% of the adolescent population [4]. The combined effects of socioeconomic status and race are clear. Disparities by race and ethnicity do exist affecting minority populations to a greater extent than majority populations [4, 29, 31]. Looking only at the adolescent population, 60% of Black adolescents and 59% of Hispanic adolescents live in low-income families. This compares with only 27% of White adolescents. Furthermore, 52% of adolescents of immigrant parents compared to 36% of adolescents of native-born parents live in low-income families [4].

The effects of poverty are complex and can have lasting effects throughout the lifespan. Two hypotheses have been proposed to account for the association between socioeconomic status and psychological problems: (a) the social causation hypothesis and (b) the social selection hypothesis [32, 33]. The social causation hypothesis postulates that psychological problems develop secondary to the adversity that the individual lives in daily. The social selection hypothesis suggests persons who have psychological concerns gradually decrease their level of income secondary to their disease creating barriers for the individual to fulfill their obligations in the expected role subsequently creating more stress creating a snowballing effect [32, 33]. These hypotheses facilitate our understanding of the many dynamics that impact the mental health status of adolescents. Low socioeconomic status often results in poor living and neighborhood conditions that often expose children to violence [27]. Other issues, including food insecurity, family mental health issues, educational opportunities, and available community resources, may contribute to the presentation and willingness to seek mental health services [31]. Adolescents living in low-income homes are at increased risk for personality disorders and depression and tend to engage in high-risk health behaviors and participate in delinquent behaviors [31, 34].

Race and Ethnicity

Although race is a social construct, US adolescents experience many racial and ethnic disparities in health and healthcare [35]. The empirical evidence suggests mental disorders disproportionally affect racial and ethnic minority youth. As previously mentioned, there are a number of ecological risk factors that impact mental disorders for all youth but in particular for racial and ethnic minority youth. A contributing factor to physical and mental health disparities in minority children may be the experiences of interpersonal and institutional racism [36, 37]. A study by Tobler et al. [37] examined the link between self-report of exposure to discrimination and its association with mental health among a sample of 2490 racial/ethnic minority adolescents primarily from low-income families. The researchers found 73% of participants reported they had experienced discrimination due to their race and/or ethnicity and 42% of those experiences were described to be somewhat disturbing or very disturbing. Findings revealed that adolescents who reported racism were more likely to exhibit aggressive behaviors, report suicide ideation, delinquency, and engage in high-risk sexual behaviors [37]. These findings also were described in a recent systemic review of the literature base (see [38]).

Due to often-reported risk factors, it is critical to engage racial and ethnic minority youth in mental health prevention and intervention strategies. However, racial and ethnic minority adolescents—like other cultural minority groups—experience disparities in access, utilization, and quality of mental health services compared to non-Hispanic White adolescents [24, 39, 40]. Racial and ethnic minorities utilize mental health services less frequently, and Black American youth are also less likely to utilize school-based and inpatient/residential mental health services than White youth [40–42]. A number of logistical barriers may influence this disparity including costs of treatment, insurance limitations, availability of treatment, and location of treatment [43]. In addition, there may be stigma-related barriers to obtaining mental health services, particularly among Hispanic and Latino families [44]. Beyond access to and utilization of mental health services, additional challenges arise from a lack of culturally competent mental health services that address adolescent needs in the context of their culture and community [45]. There is no doubt that culture influences how adolescents understand and express emotions and behaviors. Mental health practitioners who lack cultural competency and cultural humility may result in poor patient-provider communication, misunderstanding, and misdiagnosis [46, 47].

Immigrant and Refugee Populations

In the United States, new immigrant populations have unique risk factors and mental health needs. Child and adolescent refugees suffer significant conflict-related exposures [48]. Detention in refugee camps and illegal immigration increase the risk of exposure to stressors such as violence and prolonged separation from parents and caregivers [49]. Upon resettlement, in the US many individuals from these populations experience great stress related to acculturation and separation from homeland, family, and friends [48]. As a result, immigrant children often experience significant mental health symptoms and disorders: anxiety disorders, mood disorders, and posttraumatic stress disorders [49]. Like other racial, ethnic, and cultural groups, refugee and immigrant populations often underutilize mental health services due to perceived and real limited access to services and resources, stigma, low priority compared to other immediate needs, and the ability to pay [48]. Additional barriers to culturally competent care exist within the health care system. Patient navigation and linguistic and cultural understanding between patients and providers pose additional challenges [48, 49].

LGBTQQI

While adolescence is a challenging life stage for all, those who identify as lesbian, gay, bisexual, transgender, queer, questioning, or intersex (LGBTQQI) might face unique burdens of social stigma, bullying, and discrimination related to sexual orientation and gender identity [50, 51]. Thus, this population may experience additional psychological stress. Sexual minority youth also experience disproportionate victimization and exposure to adverse childhood experiences [52, 53]. As a result, they are more likely to experience psychological distress than their heterosexual counterparts [54–58]. LGBTQQI adolescents are at greater risk for poor physical and mental health and experience higher rates of depression, anxiety, conduct disorders, suicide ideation and attempts, and substance abuse or dependence [57, 59–62]. Despite the growing evidence of mental health disparities in this population, more research is needed into the health of sexual minorities, including adolescents [57, 63].

In addition to the increased risk for poor mental health in these populations, there may be additional barriers to accessing quality mental health services. Providers may be reluctant to ask about sexual orientation and gender identity, while patients can experience discomfort and fear in discussing these topics with healthcare providers [57]. Many healthcare providers lack training and understanding about the cultural and health needs of sexual minority patients and clients, which may lead to less than optimal care for LGBTQQI adolescents [57, 64]. Primary care for all adolescents should include periodic, private, and confidential discussions on a range of health issues, including sexuality and sex [64, 65].

Prevalent Mental Health Disorders in Adolescent Populations

Mental health disorders are common in adolescent populations [66]. A Centers of Disease and Prevention (CDC) review of data systems between 2013–2019 recognized the high prevalence of diagnosable mental health diseases in a younger population of 3–17 years old [66]. During the time frame, one-fifth of children in this age group had ever experienced depressive symptoms. In 2019, almost 38% of high school students experienced sadness or hopelessness, with nearly 19% seriously considering suicide [66]. The researchers reported that one in four children between the ages of 12 to 17 years had received mental health services the previous year [66]. Using data from the National Comorbidity Survey Replication Adolescent Supplement (NCS-AS) Kessler and colleagues reported the prevalence of any DSM-IV disorder in US adolescents aged 13–18 to be approximately 40% [67]. This is consistent with another study that found an estimated 46% lifetime prevalence of any mental health disorder in this age group [68]. An age gradient of risk was noted with 14–18-year olds estimated to have a 42% risk while older teens, ages 17–18 years, were found to have an approximate 54% risk of lifetime mental health illness prevalence [68]. Even more startling, lifetime prevalence of a severe mental health disorder was found to be approximately 20% or 1 in 5 children between the ages of 13 and 18 years of age [68]. Taken together, these studies point toward the high prevalence rates of mental disorders among youth in the United States.

Common disorders include both internalizing and externalizing disorders, substance abuse, and eating disorders [66–68]. In the NCS-AS study of middle and late adolescents, *anxiety disorders* were the most common diagnosis accounting for about 25–32% of mental health disorders. Within the category of anxiety disorders, *specific phobia* was the most prevalent disorder and accounted for 16–19% of the diagnoses. Despite the cause of anxiety, females account for higher lifetime rates than males. *Behavior disorders* represented the second most common type of condition at 16–19% with subcategory rates of *oppositional defiant disorder* and *attention deficit/hyperactivity* disorder (ADHD) near 8–13% and 6–9%, respectively.

Behavior disorders were more common in males compared to their female counterparts. This was closely followed by *mood disorders* with 10% to over 14% lifetime prevalence rates. Of these youth, anywhere from 8% to almost 12% were identified as having a *major depressive disorder* with almost 9% with severe disease in one study. As with anxiety disorders, mood disorders are more common in females. Additionally, the prevalence of mood disorders increases in older adolescents. Another DSM-IV disorder commonly seen in middle and late adolescents is *substance use disorders*, which were reported to range from 8% to 11% of adolescents. Lifetime prevalence rates of adolescents diagnosed with drug abuse/dependence and alcohol abuse/dependence ranged from 5% to 9%. Eating disorders affected almost 3% of adolescents. As expected these disorders (mood, anxiety, and eating disorders) increased with age and were more prevalent in females than males [68], although only a few differences were noted in regard to race and ethnicity [68]. A diagnosis of anxiety was higher among non-Hispanic Black youth compared to non-Hispanic White adolescents. Additionally, rates of mood disorders were reported more frequently for Hispanic youth than non-Hispanic youth [68]. Adolescents who belong to these cultural groups—separately and in combination—represent a vulnerable population who often fail to receive or seek out mental health services.

Adolescent Population: Under Diagnosed and Undertreated

Despite the high prevalence of mental health disorders among adolescents, there are significant barriers to culturally effective mental health services. Considering a socio-ecological perspective, the interaction of intrapersonal, interpersonal, organizational, community, and policy factors all affect mental health status, assessment, diagnosis, and treatment outcomes for adolescent populations all must be considered [5, 69]. Principally, there are many challenges in accessing adolescent mental health services. According to the National Survey of Children's Health, nearly half of *all* US adolescents lack a medical home [70] and for adolescents with mental health conditions, the rates for having a medical home are even lower [70]. Nationally, there is a shortage of providers to meet the needs of youth with mental health symptoms, and diagnoses, with even more pronounced shortages in rural and low-income communities [71]. In addition, access to adolescent mental health services varies greatly across the US as services are often dependent on state-level policies and healthcare market characteristics [72]. Thus, culturally relevant mental health services for adolescents are impacted by societal and community, familial, and individual factors.

Community-level factors such as neighborhood, socioeconomic status, social cohesion, exposure to violence, and perceived control may influence the mental health of adolescent residents [27, 73]. Butler et al. [74] found living in a neighborhood with poor physical qualities and low social support to be associated with higher odds of anxiety, depression, ADHD, and behavioral problems in adolescents, even when controlling for other neighborhood conditions, sociodemographic factors, and parental mental health. The implications of neighborhood poverty cannot be overstated [75]. Research has shown that moving from a high-poverty to low-poverty neighborhood may lead to reductions in depressive/anxiety and dependency symptoms problems in youth [76].

Other contextual and environmental factors must be considered in understanding risk pathways to adolescent health. For example, schools play an important role in adolescent mental health. Teachers and those within the school system may be the first to recognize a potential mental health problem such as disruptive behaviors or psychological distress. In fact, an individual's level of school connectedness is a significant predictor of adolescent depressive symptoms [77] and suicidality. In one recent study, high levels of school connectedness were related to low levels of suicidality among a Black adolescent sample [78]. In addition to serving as a resource and a source of support, teachers and peers can contribute to the daily stress (discrimination and bullying) experienced by adolescents as they develop and become older adolescents and emerging adults [79]. Because adolescents spend a significant time in the school environment it is important to consider how this context and adults present in the school system can exacerbate or buffer mental health outcomes [80]. School-based mental health services offer the potential for prevention efforts as well as intervention strategies, although these services are inconsistently implemented throughout the US [81].

Primary care systems are relevant to mental health detection and treatment among adolescents. Racial, ethnic, and cultural minorities are more likely to receive their mental health care (if any) from a primary care physician than a specialty provider [82]. Primary care physicians are often the sole providers of commonly prescribed medications for mental health conditions and brief office-based counseling. Thus, primary care providers must be aware of how demographic factors (age, race, gender, sexual orientation, and religion) as well as other contextual factors influence the presentation of mental health symptoms. In a review of the literature, Kohn-Wood and Hooper [46] discussed the role culturally competent primary care providers may have in decreasing mental health disparities and increasing the utilization of health care providers for mental health services specifically.

Interpersonally, parents and guardians play a significant role in identifying emotional or behavioral problems and facilitating access to mental health services [83, 84]. Differences in family structures are also linked with differences in adolescent mental health outcomes [85]. Carlson [86] reported the importance of fathers in the lives of adolescents. Active father engagement was shown to decrease aggression and antisocial behavior in some adolescents as compared to peers with less father involvement. Feelings of anxiety, depression, and low self-esteem also were reported to decrease. A family history of mental health disorders also can be implicated in adolescent mental health conditions [87]. After a review of 76 studies van Santvoort et al. [87] concluded children of parents diagnosed with a mental illness are at increased risk for the development of a mental health disorder similar to their parents.

Adolescent Population: Culturally Responsive Pediatric Care

Mental health disparities have long been discussed and empirically supported, although solutions to reduce or ameliorate these disparities have been slow to emerge. Researchers have often asserted that the prevalence of mental disorders and expression of signs and symptoms are culture-specific [88], although mental health providers and others in healthcare often lack the ability to detect, diagnose, and treat mental health disorders in adolescents in general and in racially, ethnically, and culturally diverse adolescents in particular. This lack of recognition and detection of mental disorders maintains—in part—the long-reported mental health disparities described by David Satcher in the Surgeon General's Report [89]. The lack of equal and optimal treatment for *all* adolescents remains a significant mental health and societal burden that must be addressed.

With regard to treatment, the gold standard has been to use evidence-based practices to treat mental health disorders experienced by adolescents and adults. But it remains less clear if these evidence-based practices are culturally responsive and relevant to all individuals [6]. Some researchers contend that evidence-based practices may show efficacy (i.e., the treatment works in controlled clinical trials) but fail to show effectiveness (i.e., does the treatment work in the communities where they are being practiced and with the population with whom they are being used). The Substance and Mental Health Services Administration report on the hundreds of evidence-based programs available to providers and others in the healthcare field but many of those programs may not be ecologically valid (https://www.samhsa.gov/treatment https://www.samhsa.gov/nrepp). Consequently, the mental health burden and mental health disparities often seen in the adolescent population may not be reduced even when using evidence-based practices. Hall et al. [7] suggested that treatment practices and interventions that are culturally responsive are likely to be ecologically valid and likely to reduce health disparities. An ecological mental health treatment framework would consider unique community resources, the treatment context, the cultural norms of the population, and the barriers often evidenced in the population [6].

Mental health providers and others in the healthcare field must be knowledgeable about the unique developmental, cultural, and ecological factors that impinge upon adolescent mental health outcomes and importantly barriers to treatment (e.g., treatment utilization, stigma, discrimination, geography, and health suspiciousness about treatment providers and services). In addition to this vital knowledge, mental health providers and others in the healthcare field must be competent in infusing cultural considerations into adolescent pediatric mental health care (assessment, diagnosis, and treatment). In a recent meta-analysis of cultural adaptations of mental health interventions, Hall et al. [7] documented the benefit of reducing mental health symptomatology when culturally adapted interventions were used. This research, surprisingly, is in its infancy.

Other commonly purported factors that relate to culturally responsive pediatric care and possibly related to reducing health disparities are provider cultural and linguistic competency [46, 90]. In fact, it is an ethical imperative that health providers and others in the healthcare field engage in training that facilitates cultural humility, cultural awareness, and specific knowledge and skills relevant to working with diverse adolescents and their families. In the context of office-based counseling, Cardemill and Battle [91] proffered several recommendations for providers working toward cultural competency. Their suggestions, which have transportability to all settings and most providers, include the following: (a) recognize and suspend preconceptions about patients' race, ethnicity, and other cultural identities and that of their family members, (b) recognize within differences among patients who self-identify similarly (i.e., patients may be quite different from other members of their own group), (c) consider how differences between the provider's race, ethnicity, and other cultural identities and patient's may impact the patient care process (assessment, diagnosis, and treatment), (d) recognize that discrimination, racism, power, and privilege may be implicated in the patient-provider interactions and behaviors, and (e) be prepared and willing to broach culturally related topics and their relevance to presenting issues with patients. Importantly, these recommendations may help reduce the stigma and other barriers evinced among racial, ethnic, and diverse individuals seeking services or who may terminate services prematurely.

For several decades, mental health providers and others in the healthcare field have made attempts to reduce mental health disparities with little to no success. The severe burden of undiagnosed and untreated mental health conditions among adolescents cannot be overstated. It is clear that more research is needed. More specifically, research is needed that clarifies how to successfully engage adolescents and their families in culturally responsive ways, and that elucidates what constitutes efficacious and effective ecologically valid and culturally adaptive assessment and treatment modalities for adolescent mental health conditions. Finally, as described earlier, healthcare organizational and structural "competence" are important as well. All of these dynamics are interlinked and have relevance for policy initiatives (i.e., Affordable Care Act), or potentially an alternative health system which will pave the way for more patients to receive needed services. This makes it even more essential that we have a health professional workforce who can bring different perspectives and be ready to rethink our strategies related to culturally adapted and responsive services and programs to assist in the battle against healthcare disparities. The individual (adolescent) and multiple contextual systems taken together must be considered if improvements in culturally competent pediatric care will be realized.

The most commonly used evidenced-based practices with adolescents often include cognitive behavioral therapy, interpersonal therapy, pharmacotherapy, and/or combination therapy. Although family systems therapy also is used it has less empirical support than cognitive behavioral therapy, interpersonal therapy, pharmacotherapy, and/or combination therapy. In addition, and importantly, few studies have been conducted to determine the efficacy and effectiveness of cultural adaptations of these most commonly used evidence-based treatments. Cultural adaptation has been defined as "the systematic modification of an evidence-based treatment or intervention protocol to consider language, culture, and context in such a way that it is compatible with the client's cultural patterns, meanings, and values" [92]. Although it has been purported that cultural adaptations are critical for increased positive outcomes it remains less clear what ought to be adapted and the added benefits of adaptations [93]. Thus, oftentimes clinicians must use treatments among populations for whom they were not developed, evaluated, or tested. The following treatments are some of the most widely used mental health treatments for adolescents.

Cognitive Behavior Therapy

Cognitive Behavior Therapy (CBT) is a short-term, goal-oriented therapy derived from principles of both behavioral and cognitive psychology. CBT utilizes a problem-focused strategy to develop actionable strategies to mitigate behaviors. Although CBT has been shown to be effective across the lifespan, the adolescent period presents its own unique challenges. It is imperative that the therapist takes into account the "critical developmental tasks and milestones relevant to a particular adolescent's problems (i.e., pubertal development, cognitive development, the development of behavioral autonomy, and social perspective taking during adolescence"; [94], p. 420) Holmbeck and Sharpera [95] proposed a framework to be considered when using CBT in the adolescent population. At the center of this framework is the interpersonal context of the adolescent, which takes into account the guidance of family, peers, school, and work. Interpersonal contexts are directly influenced by the primary developmental changes (i.e., biological, psychological, and social) that are occurring during adolescence. In turn, developmental outcomes of autonomy, psychosocial adjustment, and contentment with intimacy and sexuality are pursued. Mitigating all of these factors are the demographic and interpersonal characteristics, including ethnicity, family structure, gender, neighborhood, and community factors as well as socioeconomic status [94, 95]. Utilizing this framework, CBT has been shown to be effective in the treatment of adolescents with depression, anxiety, obsessive compulsive disorders (OCD), posttraumatic stress disorder (PTSD), and self-harming behaviors [96–99].

Interpersonal Psychotherapy

Interpersonal psychotherapy (IPT) is based on the theory that interpersonal conflicts or transitions maintain psychological distress. In contrast to CBT, which focuses on dysfunctional belief systems, IPT focuses on dysfunctional intercommunication processes. In addition, IPT is directed toward improving adolescents' "social problem-solving skills to increase their personal effectiveness and satisfaction with current relationships" (SAMSHA, n.d.). Although IPT is often used when adolescents present with depressive symptoms [100] it can be used for a range of mental health disorders, as well as when adolescents present with developmental issues, including discord with parents, peer relationships, problems with authority figures, and other intra- and interpersonal issues. Research shows that IPT has been culturally adapted for racially minority adolescents [101].

Family-Based Therapy

Family therapy focuses on improving the functioning of the family as a unit, or its subsystems, and/or the functioning of the individual members of the family When adolescents do access mental health services, parent and adolescent communication and interactions with providers may influence the accuracy of diagnosis, treatment plan, as well as patient compliance [83, 102]. Enhancing the communication between the different parties helps to build trust in the clinician's ability to treat the adolescent, which, in turn, provides an opportunity to develop a collaborative agreement concerning the treatment plan [102]. A collaborative approach to therapy reinforces adolescent coping skills when compliance may be hampered by known and unknown adverse effects of treatment [102]. In a review of the literature, Chovil [83] reported that utilization of the family engagement model has several benefits including advocacy on behalf of the adolescent resulting in better outcomes, increased accountability of services rendered, and providing treatment in a culturally sensitive manner. The family engagement model utilizes the ecological framework, which focuses on the family as a full partner in the care of their child. Families are empowered by building on their "strengths, capability, resiliency, and skill building…" to be actively involved in all levels of decision-making ([83], p. 9). Because many racial and ethnic minorities do not use mental health services, family engagement may not only increase service utilization but also increase effectiveness [103], although more research is needed. Other family models that have been used with culturally and racially diverse samples include structural-strategic family therapy, brief strategic family therapy, and multidimensional family therapy (see [93, 104]).

Psychopharmacology and Combination Therapy

Although medication can be beneficial for the treatment of mental health signs and symptoms and mental health disorders among adolescents, it may not always be the first-line treatment for many disorders and circumstances. In addition, many medication prescribing practices for mental health treatment in adolescents are informed by adult protocols [105]. It appears that select SSRIs (Fluoxetine and Paroxetine) and psychostimulants are the most frequently studied pharmacotherapies. Studies that have utilized pharmacotherapy in conjunction with psychotherapy have yielded positive outcomes. "The preponderance of available evidence indicates that psycho-social treatments are safer than psychoactive medications" (American Psychological Association [APA], 2006, p. 16 [106]). Finally, it is also important to note less is known about how racial and cultural factors are implicated in medication efficacy, safety, and adherence [106, 107].

Intersection of Culturally Responsive Care and the Adolescent Population—Case Study

Sharon is a 40-year-old Black American, single, heterosexual woman who has contacted a primary care physician about her oldest daughter's recent change in behavior. Specifically, her 13-year-old daughter, Brenda, has been complaining about severe headaches and stomach pains.

The mother (Sharon) is very concerned about her daughter and does not know what to do. In addition to the somatic complaints, Brenda has been very angry and irritable and has been reluctant to get up in the morning to go to school for the past few months. Also concerning, Brenda who has been a straight-A student has earned all Cs in her classes this past quarter. Brenda reports she just does not have the energy or interest to go to school. Brenda is argumentative with everyone in the family and the principal recently contacted her mother after Brenda asked to go to the nurses' office three consecutive days. During the office visit her mother, grandmother, and 6-year-old sister present to the office because they are concerned about what has been going on with Brenda. When the nurse calls Brenda back for her visit she asked that everyone stay in the waiting room so that the doctor can visit with Brenda privately.

Brenda meets with the doctor and he asked about the course of her stomach pains and headaches. He also asks about her diet and sleep routine. He notes in her chart that her BMI places her in the 95th percentile. The doctor also orders a series of tests and schedules a follow-up appointment. When Brenda leaves the exam room her mother asks to see the doctor but the nurse mentions that the doctor has ordered several tests and until the tests come back he does not have any information to share. Sharon is upset because she has no additional information but the nurse refuses to get the doctor. Because the mother had to take off from work to bring Brenda to the office, she was hoping to learn what exactly is going on with her daughter before leaving the office.

In this case, the physician appropriately assessed what was going on with Brenda physically. In particular, he focused on her most severe complaints (stomach pain and headaches) and ordered tests to see if he could better determine if something serious is going on that would require additional assessments, referrals, or pharmacotherapy.

Developmentally and Culturally Responsive Considerations

Keeping in mind the heterogeneity among racial, ethnic, and cultural groups there are a few considerations that may illustrate a culturally appropriate response and way of being for this case. Brenda presented with some common problems evidenced among adolescents in general. First, irritability is a common symptom reported by adolescents as they have everyday experiences, form peer and eventually romantic relationships, and develop a level of comfort in their school and other systems. On the other hand, the research is robust on the increase in mood disturbances during puberty for female adolescents. In this case, it appears that there may be other things going on for which the physician would want to assess (e.g., mild depression or anxiety). The somatic symptoms, coupled with irritability, lethargy, and change in grades may point to something else going on other than physical complaints, pre-diabetes or migraines. Second, in this case, it would be important to consider the extent to which cultural factors could account for Brenda's change in grades and lack of interest in going to school (e.g., discrimination, bullying, and lack of support from teachers). The physical complaints could be related to mental, social, and environmental issues. Third, the physician could benefit from including the mother and grandmother in the assessment process to clarify what they attribute to Brenda's signs and symptoms. Including the mother and grandmother could aid in learning more about the history of Brenda's presenting issues, the family history related to mental health issues, and the cultural and treatment preferences of the family. Because Brenda and the family self-identify as Black American there could be specific culturally related elements that could enhance physician-patient communications in general and for this first encounter in particular. The research suggests that oftentimes racially minority patients feel unheard and misunderstood during patient care visits. A culturally tailored approach would consider the benefits versus the limitations (adolescent privacy and autonomy) of including the mother and grandmother in the examination room [9]. A demonstration of cultural humility as the physician tries to better understand what is going on with Brenda following test results, could facilitate the patient care process (i.e., accurate assessment, diagnosis, and treatment) and lessen the chance of misdiagnosis and undertreatment. Finally, including the mother and grandmother in the first patient encounter would allow for a better understanding of potential cultural barriers and cultural factors that may be implicated in the presenting issues and treatment adherence (e.g., socioeconomic status, transportation, insurance, and treatment preferences).

Resources
- Centers for Disease Control and Prevention: Children's Mental Health.
    See: https://www.cdc.gov/childrensmentalhealth/symptoms.html
- Office of Adolescent Health.
    See: https://www.hhs.gov/ash/oah/index.html

- Substance Abuse and Mental Health Services Administration (SAMHSA): Identifying Mental Health and Substance Problems of Children and Adolescents: A Guide for Child Serving Organizations.
  See: http://store.samhsa.gov/shin/content/SMA12-4700/SMA12-4700.pdf
- Society of Clinical Child & Adolescent Psychology: Effective child therapy.
  See: http://effectivechildtherapy.org/content/ebp-options-specific-disorders
- Society for Research and Child Development.
  See: https://www.srcd.org/
- Society for Research on Adolescence.
  See: https://www.s-r-a.org/
- Eunice Kennedy Shriver National Institute of Child Health and Human Development.
  See: https://www.nichd.nih.gov/

References

1. U.S. Teen Demographics. Act for Youth. Retreived from https://actforyouth.net/adolescence/demographics.
2. Colby, S. L., & Ortman, J. M. (2015). Projections of the size and composition of the U.S. population: 2014 to 2060. Retrieved from census.gov/content/dam/Census/library/publications/2015/demo/p25-1143.pdf.
3. Johnson, K. M. & Lichter, D. L. The changing faces of America's children and youth. 2010. Retrieved from http://scholars.unh.edu/carsey/107.
4. Jiang, Y., Ekono, M., & Skinner, C.. Basic facts about low-income children: children 12 through 17 years, 2014. 2016. Retrieved from http://nccp.org/publications/pub_1147.html.
5. Hooper, L. M., & Crusto, C. A. (2013). Ecological systems theory. In K. D. Keith (Ed.), *Encyclopedia of cross-cultural psychology* (pp. 456–460). Wiley-Blackwell. https://doi.org/10.1002/9781118339893
6. Atkins, M. S., Rusch, D., Mehta, T. G., & Lakind, D. (2016). Future directions for dissemination and implementation science: aligning ecological theory and public health to close the research to practice gap. *Journal of Clinical Child & Adolescent Psychology, 45*(2), 215–226. https://doi.org/10.1080/15374416.2015.1050724. Retrieved from https://doi.org/10.1080/15374416.2015.1050724
7. Hall, G. C. N., Ibaraki, A. Y., Huang, E. R., Marti, C. N., & Stice, E. (2016). A meta-analysis of cultural adaptations of psychological interventions. *Behavior Therapy, 47*(6), 993–1014.
8. Davis, A. L. (2016). *Risk-taking behavior in adolescence: Exploring the roles of family, peers, and school.* The University of Memphis. https://www.proquest.com/docview/1885057814/fulltextPDF/19160C90071E44F4PQ/1?accountid=14665
9. Koslofsky, S., & Domenech Rodríguez, M. M. (2017). Cultural adaptations to psychotherapy: real-world applications. *Clinical Case Studies, 16*, 3–8.
10. World Health Organization. Adolescence: A period needing special attention. 2014. Retrieved from http://apps.who.int/adolescent/second-decade/section2/page3/adolescence-physical-changes.html
11. Styne, D. M. (1994). Normal and abnormal sexual development and puberty. In G. M. Besser & M. O. Thorner (Eds.), *Clinical Endocrinology* (2nd ed., pp. 13.2–13.26). Times Mirror International Publishers Limited.

12. Voutilainen, R., & Jääskeläinen, J. (2015). Premature adrenarche: Etiology, clinical findings, and consequences. *The Journal of Steroid Biochemistry and Molecular Biology, 145,* 226–236. https://doi.org/10.1016/j.jsbmb.2014.06.004
13. Rogol, A. D., Roemmich, J. N., & Clark, P. A. (2002). Growth at puberty. *The Journal of Adolescent Health, 31,* 192–200. https://doi.org/10.1016/S1054-139X(02)00485-8
14. Rogol, A. D. (2010). Sex steroids, growth hormone, leptin and the pubertal growth spurt. In S. Loche, M. Cappa, L. Ghizoni, M. Maghnie, & M. O. Savage (Eds.), *Pediatric neuroendocrinology* (pp. 77–85). Karger Publishers.
15. Bronfenbrenner, U. (1992). Ecological models on human development. In M. Gauvain & M. Cole (Eds.), *Readings on the development of children* (4th ed., pp. 3–8). Worth Publishers.
16. Erikson, E. (1998). Eight stages of man. In C. Cooper & L. Pervin (Eds.), *Personality: critical concepts in psychology* (pp. 66–77). Routledge.
17. Kohlberg, L., & Hersh, R. (1977). Moral development: a review of theory. *Theory Into Practice, 12,* 53–59. https://doi.org/10.1080/00405847709542675
18. Piaget, J. (1952). *The origins of intelligence in children.* International Universities Press.
19. Barrett, D. E. (1996). The three stages of adolescence. *The High School Journal, 79,* 333–339.
20. Spano S. Stages of adolescence development. 2004. Retrieved from http://www.human.cornell.edu/actforyouth.
21. Allen, B., & Waterman, H. (2019). *Stages of adolescence.* American Academy of Pediatrics, HealthyChildren.org. Retrieved at https://www.healthychildren.org/English/ages-stages/teen/Pages/Stages-of-Adolescence.aspx
22. Schwarz, S.W. Adolescent mental health in the United States: facts for policy makers. 2009. Retrieved from http://nccp.org/publications/pdf/text_878.pdf.
23. Warren, B. J., & Broome, B. (2011). The culture of mental illness in adolescents with urologic problems. *Urologic Nursing, 31,* 95–111.
24. Lu, W. (2019). Adolescent Depression: National Trends, Risk Factors, and Healthcare Disparities. American Journal of Health Behavior, 43(1),181–194.
25. Knight, A. M., Xie, M., & Mandell, D. S. (2016). Disparities in psychiatric diagnosis and treatment for youth with systemic lupus erythematosus: analysis of a national US medicaid sample. *The Journal of Rheumatology, 43,* 1427–1433. https://doi.org/10.3899/jrheum.150967
26. Nestor, B. A., Cheek, S. M., & Liu, R. T. (2016). Ethnic and racial differences in mental health service utilization for suicidal ideation and behavior in a nationally representative sample of adolescents. *Journal of Affective Disorders, 202,* 197–202. https://doi.org/10.1016/j.jad.2016.05.021
27. Aneshensel, C. S., & Sucoff, C. A. (1996). The neighborhood context of adolescent mental health. *Journal of Health and Social Behavior, 37,* 293–310. https://doi.org/10.2307/2137258
28. McLeod, J. D., & Shanahan, M. J. (1996). Trajectories of poverty and children's mental health. *Journal of Health and Social Behavior, 37,* 207–220. https://doi.org/10.2307/2137292
29. Hodgkinson, S., Godoy, S., Beers, L. S., & Lewin, A. (2017). Improving mental health access for low-income children and families in the primary care setting. *Pediatrics, 139,* 1–9. https://doi.org/10.1542/peds.2015-1175
30. Department of Health and Human Services. (2016). Annual update of the HHS poverty guidelines. *Federal Register, 81,* 4036–4037.
31. Trends, C. (2016). *Children in poverty: indicators on children and youth Well-being.* Child Trends Databank. Retrieved from http://www.childtrends.org/wp-content/uploads/2016/12/04_Poverty.pdf
32. van Oort, F. V., van der Ende, J., Wadsworth, M. E., Verhulst, F. C., & Achenbach, T. M. (2011). Cross-national comparison of the link between socioeconomic status and emotional and behavioral problems in youths. *Social Psychiatry and Psychiatric Epidemiology, 46,* 167–172. https://doi.org/10.1007/s00127-010-0191-5

33. Wadsworth, M. E., & Achenbach, T. M. (2005). Explaining the link between low socio-economic status and psychopathology: testing two mechanisms of the social causation hypothesis. *Journal of Consulting and Clinical Psychology, 73*, 1146–1153. https://doi.org/10.1037/0022-006X.73.6.1146

34. Voisin, D. R., Elsaesser, C., Ha Kim, D., Patel, S., & Cantara, A. (2016). The relationship between family stress and behavioral health among African American adolescents. *Journal of Child and Family Studies, 25*, 2201–2210. https://doi.org/10.1007/s10826-016-0402-0

35. Lau, M., Lin, H., & Flores, G. (2012). Racial/ethnic disparities in health and health care among U.S. adolescents. *Health Services Research, 47*, 2031–2059. https://doi.org/10.1111/j.1475-6773.2012.01394.x

36. Acevedo-Garcia, D., Rosenfeld, L. E., Hardy, E., McArdle, N., & Osypuk, T. L. (2013). Future directions in research on institutional and interpersonal discrimination and children's health. *American Journal of Public Health, 103*, 1754–1763. https://doi.org/10.2105/ajph.2012.300986

37. Tobler, A. L., Maldonado-Molina, M. M., Staras, S. A., O'Mara, R. J., Livingston, M. D., & Komro, K. A. (2013). Perceived racial/ethnic discrimination, problem behaviors, and mental health among minority urban youth. *Ethnicity & Health, 18*, 337–349. https://doi.org/10.1080/13557858.2012.730609

38. Priest, N., Paradies, Y., Trenerry, B., Truong, M., Karlsen, S., & Kelly, Y. (2013). A systematic review of studies examining the relationship between reported racism and health and well-being for children and young people. *Social Science & Medicine, 95*, 115–127. https://doi.org/10.1016/j.socscimed.2012.11.031

39. Alegria, M., Vallas, M., & Pumariega, A. J. (2010). Racial and ethnic disparities in pediatric mental health. *Child and Adolescent Psychiatric Clinics of North America, 19*, 759–774. https://doi.org/10.1016/j.chc.2010.07.001

40. Institute of Medicine. (2003). *Unequal treatment: confronting racial and ethnic disparities in health care*. National Academies Press.

41. Institute of Medicine. (2009). *Focusing on children's health: community approaches to addressing health disparities*. National Academies Press.

42. Barksdale, C. L., Azur, M., & Leaf, P. J. (2010). Differences in mental health service sector utilization among African American and Caucasian youth entering systems of care programs. *The Journal of Behavioral Health Services & Research, 37*, 363–373. https://doi.org/10.1007/s11414-009-9166-2

43. Thurston, I. B., & Phares, V. (2008). Mental health service utilization among African American and Caucasian mothers and fathers. *Journal of Consulting and Clinical Psychology, 76*, 1058–1067. https://doi.org/10.1037/a0014007

44. Young, A. S., & Rabiner, D. (2015). Racial/ethnic differences in parent-reported barriers to accessing children's health services. *Psychological Services, 12*, 267–273. https://doi.org/10.1037/a0038701

45. Pumariega, A. J., Rogers, K., & Rothe, E. (2005a). Culturally competent systems of care for children's mental health: advances and challenges. *Community Mental Health Journal, 41*, 539–555. https://doi.org/10.1007/s10597-005-6360-4

46. Kohn-Wood, L., & Hooper, L. M. (2014). Cultural competency, culturally tailored care, and the primary care setting: possible solutions to reduce racial/ethnic disparities in mental health care. *Journal of Mental Health Counseling, 36*, 173–188. https://doi.org/10.17744/mehc.36.2.d73h217l81tg6uv3

47. Cooper, L. A., Roter, D. L., Johnson, R. L., Ford, D. E., Steinwachs, D. M., & Powe, N. R. (2003). Patient-centered communication, ratings of care, and concordance of patient and physician race. *Annals of Internal Medicine, 139*, 907–915.

48. Lustig, S. L., Kia-Keating, M., Knight, W. G., Geltman, P., Ellis, H., Kinzie, J. D., et al. (2004). Review of child and adolescent refugee mental health. *Journal of the American Academy of Child and Adolescent Psychiatry, 43*, 24–36. https://doi.org/10.1097/00004583-200401000-00012

49. Pumariega, A. J., Rothe, E., & Pumariega, J. B. (2005b). Mental health of immigrants and refugees. *Community Mental Health Journal, 41*, 581–597. https://doi.org/10.1007/s10597-005-6363-1

50. Diaz, R. M., Ayala, G., Bein, E., Henne, J., & Marin, B. V. (2001). The impact of homophobia, poverty, and racism on the mental health of gay and bisexual Latino men: findings from 3 US cities. *American Journal of Public Health, 91*, 927–932.

51. Martin-Storey, A., Cheadle, J. E., Skalamera, J., & Crosnoe, R. (2015). Exploring the social integration of sexual minority youth across high school contexts. *Child Development, 86*, 965–975. https://doi.org/10.1111/cdev.12352

52. McLaughlin, K. A., Hatzenbuehler, M. L., Xuan, Z., & Conron, K. J. (2012). Disproportionate exposure to early-life adversity and sexual orientation disparities in psychiatric morbidity. *Child Abuse & Neglect, 36*, 645–655. https://doi.org/10.1016/j.chiabu.2012.07.004

53. Russell, S. T., Franz, B. T., & Driscoll, A. K. (2001). Same-sex romantic attraction and experiences of violence in adolescence. *American Journal of Public Health, 91*, 903–906.

54. Hatzenbuehler, M. L. (2011). The social environment and suicide attempts in lesbian, gay, and bisexual youth. *Pediatrics, 127*, 896–903. https://doi.org/10.1542/peds.2010-3020

55. Mays, V. M., & Cochran, S. D. (2001). Mental health correlates of perceived discrimination among lesbian, gay, and bisexual adults in the United States. *American Journal of Public Health, 91*, 1869–1876. https://doi.org/10.2105/AJPH.91.11.1869

56. Hatzenbuehler, M. L., McLaughlin, K. A., Keyes, K. M., & Hasin, D. S. (2010). The impact of institutional discrimination on psychiatric disorders in lesbian, gay, and bisexual populations: a prospective study. *American Journal of Public Health, 100*, 452–459. https://doi.org/10.2105/AJPH.2009.168815

57. Institute of Medicine. (2011). *The health of lesbian, gay, bisexual, and transgender people: building a foundation for better understanding* (Vol. 10, p. 13128). Institute of Medicine. Retrieved from https://www.nap.edu/read/13128/chapter/1

58. McLaughlin, K. A., & Hatzenbuehler, M. L. (2009). Mechanisms linking stressful life events and mental health problems in a prospective, community-based sample of adolescents. *The Journal of Adolescent Health, 44*, 153–160. https://doi.org/10.1016/j.jadohealth.2008.06.019

59. Marshal, M. P., King, K. M., Stepp, S. D., Hipwell, A., Smith, H., Chung, T., et al. (2012). Trajectories of alcohol and cigarette use among sexual minority and heterosexual girls. *The Journal of Adolescent Health, 50*, 97–99. https://doi.org/10.1016/j.jadohealth.2011.05.008

60. Fergusson, D. M., Horwood, L. J., & Beautrais, A. L. (1999). Is sexual orientation related to mental health problems and suicidality in young people? *Archives of General Psychiatry, 56*, 876–880. https://doi.org/10.1001/archpsyc.56.10.876

61. Levine, D. A. (2013). Office-based care for lesbian, gay, bisexual, transgender, and questioning youth. *Pediatrics, 132*, e297–e313. https://doi.org/10.1542/peds.2013-1283

62. Strutz, K. L., Herring, A. H., & Halpern, C. T. (2015). Health disparities among young adult sexual minorities in the U.S. *American Journal of Preventive Medicine, 48*(1), 76–88. https://doi.org/10.1016/j.amepre.2014.07.038

63. Mustanski, B. (2015). Future directions in research on sexual minority adolescent mental, behavioral, and sexual health. *Journal of Clinical Child and Adolescent Psychology, 44*, 204–219. https://doi.org/10.1080/15374416.2014.982756

64. Coker, T. R., Austin, S. B., & Schuster, M. A. (2010). The health and health care of lesbian, gay, and bisexual adolescents. *Annual Review of Public Health, 31*, 457–477. https://doi.org/10.1146/annurev.publhealth.012809.103636

65. Frankowski, B. L., & American Academy of Pediatrics Committee on Adolescence. (2004). Sexual orientation and adolescence. *Pediatrics, 113*, 1827–1832.

66. Bitsko, R. H., Claussen, A. H., Lichstein, J., et al. (2022). Mental health surveillance among children—United States, 2013–2019. *MMWR Supplements, 71*(Suppl-2), 1–42. https://doi.org/10.15585/mmwr.su7102a1

67. Kessler, R. C., Avenevoli, S., Costello, E. J., Georgiades, K., Green, J. G., Gruber, M. J., et al. (2012). Prevalence, persistence, and sociodemographic correlates of DSM-IV disorders in

the National Comorbidity Survey Replication Adolescent Supplement. *Archives of General Psychiatry, 69*, 372–380. https://doi.org/10.1001/archgenpsychiatry.2011.160

68. Merikangas, K. R., He, J. P., Burstein, M., Swanson, S. A., Avenevoli, S., Cui, L., et al. (2010). Lifetime prevalence of mental disorders in US adolescents: results from the National Comorbidity Survey Replication–Adolescent Supplement (NCS-A). *Journal of the American Academy of Child and Adolescent Psychiatry, 49*, 980–989. https://doi.org/10.1016/j.jaac.2010.05.017

69. McLeroy, K. R., Bibeau, D., Steckler, A., & Glanz, K. (1988). An ecological perspective on health promotion programs. *Health Education & Behavior, 15*, 351–377. https://doi.org/10.1177/109019818801500401

70. Adams, S. H., Newacheck, P. W., Park, M. J., Brindis, C. D., & Irwin, C. E. (2013). Medical home for adolescents: low attainment rates for those with mental health problems and other vulnerable groups. *Academic Pediatrics, 13*, 113–121. https://doi.org/10.1016/j.acap.2012.11.004

71. Thomas, C. R., & Holzer, C. E. (2006). The continuing shortage of child and adolescent psychiatrists. *Journal of the American Academy of Child and Adolescent Psychiatry, 45*, 1023–1031. https://doi.org/10.1097/01.chi.0000225353.16831.5d

72. Sturm, R., Ringel, J. S., & Andreyeva, T. (2003). Geographic disparities in children's mental health care. *Pediatrics, 112*, e308–e315. https://doi.org/10.1542/peds.112.4.e308

73. Donnelly, L., McLanahan, S., Brooks-Gunn, J., Garfinkel, I., Wagner, B. C., Jacobsen, W. C., et al. (2016). Cohesive Neighborhoods where social expectations are shared may have positive impact on adolescent mental health. *Health Affairs, 35*, 2083–2091.

74. Butler, A. M., Kowalkowski, M., Jones, H. A., & Raphael, J. L. (2012). The relationship of reported neighborhood conditions with child mental health. *Academic Pediatrics, 12*, 523–531. https://doi.org/10.1016/j.acap.2012.06.005

75. Bolland, J. M. (2003). Hopelessness and risk behaviour among adolescents living in high-poverty inner-city neighbourhoods. Journal of Adolescence, 26, 145–158. https://doi.org/10.1016/S0140-1971(02)00136-7.

76. Leventhal, T., & Brooks-Gunn, J. (2003). Moving to opportunity: an experimental study of neighborhood effects on mental health. *American Journal of Public Health, 93*, 1576–1582. https://doi.org/10.2105/AJPH.93.9.1576

77. Shochet, I. M., Dadds, M. R., Ham, D., & Montague, R. (2006). School connectedness is an underemphasized parameter in adolescent mental health: results of a community prediction study. *Journal of Clinical Child and Adolescent Psychology, 35*, 170–179. https://doi.org/10.1207/s15374424jccp3502_1

78. Tomek, S., Burton, S., Hooper, L. M., et al. (2018). Suicidality in Black American youth living in impoverished neighborhoods: is school connectedness a protective factor? *School Mental Health, 10*, 1–11. https://doi.org/10.1007/s12310-017-9241-4

79. Cogburn, C. D., Chavous, T. M., & Griffin, T. M. (2011). School-based racial and gender discrimination among African American adolescents: exploring gender variation in frequency and implications for adjustment. *Race and Social Problems, 3*, 25–37. https://doi.org/10.1007/s12552-011-9040-8

80. Rutter, M. (1982). *Fifteen thousand hours: secondary schools and their effects on children.* Harvard University Press.

81. Committee on School Health. (2004). School-based mental health services. *Pediatrics, 113*, 1839–1845.

82. Pingitore, D., Snowden, L., Sansone, R. A., & Klinkman, M. (2001). Persons with depressive symptoms and the treatments they receive: a comparison of primary care physicians and psychiatrists. *The International Journal of Psychiatry in Medicine, 31*, 41–60.

83. Chovil, N. (2009). Engaging families in child & youth mental health: a review of best, emerging and promising practices. *The FORCE Society for Kids' Mental Health, 20*, 26. Retrieved from   http://www.forcesociety.com/sites/default/files/Engaging%20Families%20in%20Child%20&%20Youth%20Mental%20Health.pdf

84. Logan, D. E., & King, C. A. (2001). Parental facilitation of adolescent mental health service utilization: a conceptual and empirical review. *Clinical Psychology: Science and Practice, 8,* 319–333. https://doi.org/10.1093/clipsy.8.3.319

85. Langton, C. E., & Berger, L. M. (2011). Family structure and adolescent physical health, behavior, and emotional Well-being. *The Social Service Review, 85,* 323–357. https://doi.org/10.1086/661922

86. Carlson, M. J. (2006). Family structure, father involvement, and adolescent behavioral outcomes. *Journal of Marriage and the Family, 68,* 137–154. https://doi.org/10.1111/j.1741-3737.2006.00239.x

87. van Santvoort, F., Hosman, C. M., Janssens, J. M., van Doesum, K. T., Reupert, A., & van Loon, L. M. (2015). The impact of various parental mental disorders on children's diagnoses: a systematic review. *Clinical Child and Family Psychology Review, 18,* 281–299. https://doi.org/10.1007/s10567-015-0191-9

88. Kagawa-Singer, M., Dressler, W. W., George, S. M., & Ellwood, W. M. (2015). *The cultural framework for health: an integrative approach for research and program design and evaluation.* National Institutes of Health.

89. Department of Health and Human Services. U.S. Public Health Service. Mental Health: a Report of the Surgeon General. (1999) Retrieved from https://profiles.nlm.nih.gov/spotlight/nn/catalog/nlm:nlmuid-101584932X120-doc

90. Betancourt, J. R., Green, A. R., Carrillo, J. E., & Ananeh-Firempong, O. (2003). Defining cultural competence: a practical framework for addressing racial/ethnic disparities in health and health care. *Public Health Reports, 118,* 293–302.

91. Cardemil, E. V., & Battle, C. L. (2003). Guess who's coming to therapy? Getting comfortable with conversations about race and ethnicity in psychotherapy. *Professional Psychology: Research and Practice, 34*(3), 278–286. Copyright 2003 by the American Psychological Association, Inc. 2003. Retrieved from https://citeseerx.ist.psu.edu/document?repid=rep1&type=pdf&doi=ca97e00e9182b30fd21692474c84197ba885f011

92. Bernal, G., & Jimenez-Chafey, M. I. (2009). Cultural adaptations of treatments: A resource for considering culture in evidence-based practice. *Professional Psychiatry: Research and Practice, 40*(4), 361–368. https://doi.org/10.1037/a0016401

93. Huey, S. J., & Polo, A. J. (2008). Evidence-based psychosocial treatments for ethnic minority youth. *Journal of Clinical Child and Adolescent Psychology, 37,* 262–301.

94. Holmbeck, G. N., O'Mahar, K., Abad, M., Colder, C., & Updegrove, A. (2006). Cognitive-behavioral therapy with adolescents. In P. C. Kendall (Ed.), *Child and adolescent therapy* (3rd ed., pp. 419–464). The Guilford Press.

95. Holmbeck, G. N., & Shapera, W. F. (1999). Research methods with adolescents. In P. C. Kendall, J. N. Butcher, & G. N. Holmbeck (Eds.), *Handbook of research methods in clinical psychology* (2nd ed., pp. 634–661). Wiley.

96. van Starrenburg, M. L., Kuijpers, R. C., Kleinjan, M., Hutschemaekers, G. J., & Engels, R. C. (2017). Effectiveness of cognitive behavioral therapy-based indicated prevention program for children with elevated anxiety levels: a randomized controlled trial. *Prevention Science, 18,* 31–39. https://doi.org/10.1007/s11121-016-0725-5

97. Brown, A., Creswell, C., Barker, C., Bulter, S., Cooper, P., Hobbs, C., & Thirlwall, K. (2017). Guided parent-delivered cognitive behaviour therapy for children with anxiety disorders: outcomes at 3-to 5-year follow-up. *The British Journal of Clinical Psychology, 2,* 149–159. https://doi.org/10.1111/bjc.12127

98. Spirito, A., Esposito-Smythers, C., Wolff, J., & Uhl, K. (2011). Cognitive-behavioral therapy for adolescent depression and suicidality. *Child and Adolescent Psychiatric Clinics of North America, 20,* 191–204. https://doi.org/10.1016/j.chc.2011.01.012

99. Munoz-Solomando, A., Kendell, T., & Whittington, C. J. (2008). Cognitive behavioral therapy for children and adolescents. *Current Opinion in Psychiatry, 21,* 332–337. https://doi.org/10.1097/YCO.0b013e328305097c

100. Mufson, L., Dorta, K. P., Wickramaratne, P., Nomura, Y., Olfson, M., & Weissman, M. M. (2004). A randomized effectiveness trial of interpersonal psychotherapy for depressed adolescents. *Archives of General Psychiatry, 61*(6), 577–584.
101. Rosselló, J., Bernal, G., & Rivera-Medina, C. (2012). *Individual and group CBT and IPT for Puerto Rican adolescents with depressive symptoms.* Journal of Latina/o Psychology Advance online publication.
102. Staton, D. (2010). Achieving adolescent adherence to treatment of major depression. *Adolescent Health, Medicine and Therapeutics, 1,* 73–85. https://doi.org/10.2147/AHMT.S8791
103. Spencer, S. A., Blau, G. M., & Mallery, C. J. (2010). Family-driven care in america: more than a good idea. *Journal of the Canadian Academy of Child and Adolescent Psychiatry, 19*(3), 176–181. PMID: 20842272; PMCID: PMC2938750.
104. Szapocznik, J., & Williams, R. A. (2000). Brief strategic family therapy: twenty-five years of interplay among theory, research and practice in adolescent behavior problems and drug abuse. *Clinical Child and Family Psychology Review, 3,* 117–134.
105. Hoagwood, K., Burns, B. J., Kiser, L., Ringeisen, H., & Schoenwald, S. K. (2001). Evidence-based practice in child and adolescent mental health services. *Psychiatric Services, 52,* 1179–1189.
106. American Psychological Association. (2006). *APA working group on psychoactive medications for children and adolescents* (Report of the working group on psychoactive medications for children and adolescents: psychopharmacological, psychosocial, and combined interventions for childhood disorders: evidence base, contextual factors, and future directions). American Psychological Association.
107. McQuaid, E. L., & Landier, W. (2018). Cultural issues in medication adherence: Disparities and directions. *Journal of General Internal Medicine, 33*(2), 200–206. https://doi.org/10.1007/s11606-017-4199-3. PMID: 29204971; PMCID: PMC5789102.

V. Faye Jones, M.D., Ph.D., M.S.P.H. serves as the Associate Vice President for Health Affairs/Diversity Initiatives for the Health Science Center Campus and Vice Chair in the Department of Pediatrics at the University of Louisville School of Medicine. She has been in academia for 33 years and a practicing general pediatrician for 35 years.

Katie F. Leslie, Ph.D., M.S. is an Associate Professor in the Department of Pharmacy Practice and currently serves as Director of Enrollment and Community Outreach for Sullivan University College of Pharmacy and Health Sciences in Louisville, KY. Dr. Leslie was a former professional with the University of Louisville.

Lisa M. Hooper, Ph.D. is Professor and Richard O. Jacobson Endowed Chair and Director Center for Educational Transformation Research at the University of Northern Iowa Center for Educational Transformation. She formerly served as faculty at the University of Louisville in Louisville, KY.

Chapter 3
Treatment of Women in Healthcare Environments

Monica D. Griffin and Idella G. Glenn

Women consumers of healthcare in the United States comprise a distinctly vulnerable population within every sector of healthcare, including pharmaceutical medicine, insurance coverage, and disparity outcomes. Poor women of color are at a demonstrated disadvantage in maintaining good health and longevity [1]. Medical professionals and staff are challenged to meet the diverse health needs of patients in environments that are sustained by the efficiency of standardized, technology-based means of assessment and then treatment [2]. But how? Medical professionals extend treatment amid pressures of efficiency and the myriad circumstances presented by patients across intersections of race, class, and gender (among other social identity categories); leading health research recommendations on competent approaches to treatment also reflect these challenges (see [3]; Togami et al. 2018). Toward the goal of deepening our understanding of women's treatment as patients, this chapter uses a pilot survey of providers' perceptions about women's healthcare experiences to explore themes in the literature about women's differential health outcomes and their encounters in healthcare systems in order to imagine providers' roles as pivotal in managing improvement toward better health.

Twentieth century US medicine underwent a social transformation of professionalization that social historian Paul Starr [4] called *medicalization* which involved a significant process of reorganization in terms of recognizing particular social and cultural institutions, organizations, and practices as legitimate for identifying, treating, and understanding human health [4]. Twenty-first century social

M. D. Griffin (✉)
Charles Center, William and Mary, Williamsburg, VA, USA
e-mail: mdgrif@wm.edu

I. G. Glenn
Equity and Inclusion—Office of the President, University of Southern Maine, Portland, ME, USA

transformations in medicine are described by Clarke et al. [5] as *biomedicalization*—a complex set of social interactions, transactions, and meanings that occur within the presently advanced technological and scientific industries of US medicine, furthermore shaped by pharmaceutical, information, and bio-cellular markets for advancing human health and knowledge about health [5].

In the writing of this chapter, in the context of the COVID-19 pandemic, the complexity of twenty-first century healthcare as a practice cannot be overstated. Global stakeholders recognized crosscutting global health threats ranging from "antimicrobial resistance, pollution, food security, biosafety, biosecurity, and emerging and reemerging infectious diseases" prior to the COVID-19 outbreak, issuing a call for the United States to develop a more formal version of a "transdisciplinary approach" to medical science and treatment that builds extensively on the Institute of Medicine's (IOM's) [3] 5 Core Competencies in an effort to advance medical education and training (Togami et al. 2018; IOM [3]). To summarize, the IOM Core Competencies that health clinicians "regardless of their discipline" need to undertake are: (1) to provide patient-centered care, (2) to work in interdisciplinary teams, (3) to employ evidence-based practice, (4) to apply quality improvement, and (5) to utilize informatics (IOM, [3]).

Models of healthcare treatment remain abstract, and often removed from the experiences of patients without evaluative and qualitative assessments of practice. McDermott et al. (2019) demonstrates that medical students can grow in their professional identities and participate as change agents, even within the complicated contexts of current medicine in their case summary research. They argue for continuing transformation in medication education as a step toward improved health practice and outcomes:

> As health systems are adapting to increased accountability for quality outcomes, population health, and collaborative care, medical schools are adapting curricula to better prepare physicians to function in health systems. Two components of this educational transformation are (1) increasing physician competence in Health Systems Science, including quality, population health, social determinants of health, and interprofessional collaboration, and (2) providing roles for students to act as change agents while adding value to the health system.

Specifically, the authors use three (3) case summaries (from their own medical training experiences) to describe activities and insights they gained from the practical experience of *patient navigation*. *Patient navigation* refers to "intervention using outreach workers to assess barriers to care and assist patients in navigating complex healthcare systems to optimize care and reduce disparities." McDermott et al. (2019) demonstrates persuasively the continuing significance of the medical encounter as a time-and-space site for healthcare professionals to gain insights about care, particularly in areas of improving a patient's medical care, improving a clinic's care and improving transparency of health system resources. Notably, their time- and setting-specific observations of gaps in care replicate the IOM's five competencies and the concerns of global stakeholders who developed the One Health transdisciplinary approach to medical treatment, specifically in the competency domains of "leadership," "systems thinking," and "communication and informatics" (Togami et al.

2018). McDermott et al.'s (2019) research demonstrates the potential for small-scale, qualitative research to inform practitioners of patient-centered care within contemporary healthcare systems that involve a range of factors in human behavior, communication, and information management.

This research aims to add to the understanding of women's health disparities in medical research scholarship the perceptions medical practitioners as a way to engage the capacity of medical professionals' roles for making important observations and using professional agency to improve the quality of women's healthcare. Our review of the literature reveals important trends in women's healthcare, in terms of the quality of care, access to care, women's perceptions of providers, biases in women's treatment, and specific services for women—themes that we used to inform the study summarized below. Providers' perceptions of women's treatment in medicine allow us to explore the value of a mixed methods approach to medical research (and practice) in women's health and to assess the feasibility of a larger scale, qualitative investigation as warranted. The authors agree that the predominant reliance on population data analysis, aggregate health outcomes research, and particular sciences research offers valuable information about human health, and women's health in particular; but we argue that health providers can gain much more knowledge by triangulating big data in health with qualitative, region-, and community-based research as they seek to improve the quality of care, they offer patients in their clinics and regions.

The present study uses a qualitative questionnaire to investigate: Do practitioners recognize and/or agree with the significant areas of healthcare that impact women's health experiences identified by the scholarship? And if so, in what ways? If not, why (do they suppose)? Specifically, we wanted to know

1. Do practitioners recognize areas of healthcare that impact women's health experiences that are not identified in our review of current scholarship? If so, what are they?
2. Are there specific ways in which practitioners can adjust or intervene to improve women's treatment in healthcare in any of these areas?

Themes in Research on Women's Treatment in Healthcare

Scholarship on women's treatment as patients relies heavily on population data, both qualitative and quantitative surveys of patient experiences and policy analysis. Our review found that much of the research about women's treatment in healthcare environments focused on health outcomes, as impacted by social determinants of health, and varied by demographic variables such as race, age, and gender, or by income level or income inequality in a region. Health disparities and intersectional effects between variables were further indicated in the literature, in terms of population data and health outcomes such as disease prevalence, longevity, or morbidity. Furthermore, women's health literature predictably spanned a range of themes that addressed the dynamic social processes of healthcare delivery within a recognizably complex market of clinical and treatment encounters. Several themes emerge in scholarship on women's treatment as patients in healthcare, apart from epidemiological findings in health disparities: (a) quality of healthcare; (b) limited access to adequate healthcare; (c) women's perceptions of providers; (d) experience of bias; (e) the roles women play as consumers and advocates; and (f) healthcare services that are specific to women.

Quality of Care

In 2011, the Agency for Healthcare Research and Quality reported on four emerging themes in healthcare disparities for women that emphasize the need to accelerate progress if the nation is to achieve higher quality and more equitable healthcare:

1. Healthcare quality and access are suboptimal, especially for minority and low-income groups. For example, "women age 40 and over who reported they had a mammogram within 2 years was 67.1% in 2008, slightly up from 66.6% in 2005; the rate of breast cancer deaths per 100,000 women was 22.9% in 2007, 23.5% in 2006, and 24.1% in 2005."
2. Quality is improving, but access and disparities are not improving. Examples: "from 1999–2001 to 2005–2007, males and females had significant decreases in the hospitalization for lower extremity amputation; in 2008 the percentage of female adult hemodialysis patients receiving adequate dialysis was higher than that of males."
3. Urgent attention is warranted to ensure improvements in quality and progress in reducing disparities with respect to certain services, geographic areas, and population. These should include:

   (a) cancer screening and management of diabetes,
   (b) states in the central part of the country,
   (c) residents in inner-city and rural areas,
   (d) disparities in preventive services and access to care.

4. Progress is uneven with respect to eight national priority areas:

   (a) two are improving in quality: palliative and end-of-life care and patient and family engagement,
   (b) three are lagging: population, health, safety, and access,
   (c) three require more data to assess: care coordination, overuse, and health system infrastructure,
   (d) all eight priorities showed disparities related to race, ethnicity, and socioeconomic status [6].

Key findings from the 2018 National Healthcare Quality and Disparities (NHQD) Report indicate that between 2000 and 2017, 50% of healthcare access measures showed improvement, 33% showed no improvement, and 14% showed worsening. Researchers attribute significant gains to improvement in health insurance coverage for the general population. Researchers' findings in terms of quality of care are summarized below, by identified priorities:

- *Person-Centered Care*: Almost 70% of person-centered care measures were improving overall.
- *Patient Safety*: More than 60% of patient safety measures were improving overall.
- *Healthy Living*: Almost 60% of healthy living measures were improving overall.
- *Effective Treatment*: Almost half of the effective treatment measures were improving overall.
- *Care Coordination*: One-third of care coordination measures were improving overall.
- *Care Affordability*: No care affordability measures have changed overall.

NHQD Researchers noted that "[o]verall, some disparities were getting smaller from 2000 through 2016–2017, but disparities persist, especially for poor and uninsured populations in all priority areas."

Lack of Access to Healthcare

US health insurance operates through for-profit corporations that broker with employers, medical associations, pharmaceutical companies, investors, and others, to leverage costs in extending the opportunity for preventive medicine, treatments, and acute health needs [5]. Individuals are typically covered through their employers, on their own through a private corporation, or through a spouse's or parent's similarly brokered system. Some people are covered through public assistance or policies under the Affordable Care Act (ACA), which has undergone several problematic iterations in determining what it covers, whom it covers, and for how much.

In a study comparing men's and women's access to healthcare, Merzel [7] found (in a community sample of 695 urban participants) that no strong pattern emerges to explain gender differentials in having insurance coverage and having a primary care provider. Women who were employed were more likely to have insurance coverage. However, employment did not have a similar effect on men's insurance coverage. Socioeconomic factors were important determinants of having a steady source of coverage for men, but "public assistance evidenced a strong relationship with insurance coverage among both men and women" [7]. Researchers concluded that public assistance and affordable health coverage would go far in reducing gender disparities in health, especially in low-income communities [7].

The Affordable Care Act (ACA) passed in 2010 required that most individuals have some type of health coverage by 2014. While many women (58%) are covered by their employer-sponsored insurance many are exposed to losing coverage because women are twice as likely to be covered as a dependent thus making them vulnerable should they become widowed, divorced, or spouse loses a job [8]. Of those who are uninsured (20%) the majority are low income or poor.

Women's Perception of Providers

Women's perceptions of providers matter, especially since they take on primary roles as seekers of healthcare within households [9]. This chapter's authors found women's perceptions of providers to be prevalent in the literature, a complex phenomenon mediated by several factors that included both patients' and providers' behaviors. Studies reveal consistently that women's perceptions of providers were often indicated by their choices in the types of medical treatment or advice they seek, compliance with medical advice, and that satisfaction with their experiences varied in ways that offer insight for responsiveness or intervention on the part of providers [9]. For example, Bronstein et al. [10] found that "more than half (56%) of [women clients] reported having one or more general health concerns" beyond noncontraceptive health concerns when seeking treatment through a family planning provider. In other words, women are choosing to seek general and primary healthcare in settings designed for gynecological, or reproductive medicine treatment. Women's health behavior, in seeking treatment, identifying settings for treatment, compliance with medical advice, and satisfaction—all suggest that contexts of care may indicate that a complex approach to studying the quality of care in women's health is warranted, beyond assessments that are revealed by population data reporting.

Salmon [11] examined women's perception of healthcare providers, social support, and program support in an outpatient drug treatment program [11]. Data was collected through a demographic questionnaire and a tool designed by the authors based on the Social Stress Model for Substance Abuse and the literature on social support. Most of the women in the study were satisfied with their social support from family and friends. However, 66% of the women felt that the support received from medical providers was not adequate, though. Also, according to the study, most women received no information on the risks of drug use during pregnancy from their medical providers (p. 245). Nevertheless, the women felt the program helped maintain abstinence by providing education, coping mechanism, resources, 12-step programs, and spiritual guidance. Findings suggest that reproductive healthcare nurse practitioners and physicians need to communicate the risks of substance abuse and pregnancy with their clients, more clearly if already doing so. The study demonstrates overlapping areas of healthcare that are particular to women's life circumstances and warrant qualitative attention in the content of provider–patient interaction, as much as the systems level of clinical care and coordination.

Patients' expectations for clinical care can impact health behavior, outcomes, and satisfaction with services too. Guiahi et al. [12] developed a study to determine if women anticipate a difference in reproductive care when attending a Catholic hospital. The study of what women anticipate in healthcare also reveals where gaps in care, transparency, and practice may exist. The study asserts that the "Catholic church exerts major influence over the United States healthcare system by oversee-ing the largest group of not-for-profit healthcare sponsors, systems, and facilities. As of 2011, 10% of all acute-care hospitals were Catholic sponsored or affiliated" [12]. In the study, women were randomized to hypothetical women's health clinics at either a secular or Catholic hospital and asked about expectations for family plan-ning care. Two hundred and thirty six surveys were completed with most of the participants identifying as young, white, non-Hispanic, single women who have never been pregnant. The most commonly identified religion was either agnostic/atheist/no religion, and the majority had completed an undergraduate or gradu-ate degree.

Many of the participants expected their gynecologist to provide all family plan-ning services presented [12]. The only difference based on institution was that par-ticipants randomized to the Catholic hospital were more likely to expect natural family planning advice. At least half of respondents reported they would seek care from their gynecologist for the services surveyed with the exceptions of emergency contraception and elective abortion. This cohort of women did not anticipate differ-ences in reproductive healthcare based on institution. Guiahi et al. [12] note "when women are cared for at Catholic owned hospitals, they face several restrictions to reproductive healthcare, including access to birth control methods, emergency con-traception, and miscarriage management." But if women enrolled at Catholic hospi-tals do not receive information related to potential healthcare restrictions, their ability to act as informed healthcare consumers may be constrained. Additionally, Guiahi et al. [12] point out that obstetrician-gynecologists who practice at reli-giously affiliated hospitals have reported conflicts with religious policies for patient care. Each study presents the question qualitatively: what mediating factors might occur in any clinical setting to impact women's treatment in health negatively or positively?

Trentalange et al. [13] conducted a national patient experience survey, adminis-tered to 720 women veterans, in order to examine their perceptions of providers, in accounting for women's satisfaction in their encounters with designated women's health providers (DWHPs) as compared with non-DWHPs or nurse practitioners. In addition to studying women's perceptions of providers, the authors aimed to add understanding to how mediating factors of the medical encounter shaped satisfac-tion with outcomes. According to Trentalange et al. [13] several factors might inform a patient's perception of a provider, such as time spent with a patient or how much a provider exceeded or met a patient's expectations for the visit. Trentalange et al. [13] note a variety of examples from Weiss' [14] research, regarding *how* patient perceptions of enough time can be influenced:

> Patient perceptions of enough time is subjective and can be influenced by provider behavior and communication style such as use of eye contact, voice tone, pace of speech, and choice of topics to be discussed during the visit. For example, how fast a provider speaks can either strengthen or diminish the patient's sense that their provider is spending enough time addressing their needs [14]

Trentalange [13] found that "[r]elative to other patients, those seen by nurse practitioners or DWHPs exhibit overall satisfaction that is, on average, about 3% higher or 0.3 on a 10-point scale" (Trentalage 2016). The findings show that "neither provider class nor provider designation exhibit significant direct associations with overall satisfaction"; instead, in their estimation, "80% of the respective associations between provider class and provider designation can be attributed to [a mediating factor such as] patient perception of enough time spent by the provider [13]. This study suggests that neither patient expectations of a clinical visit nor the particular provider class have a direct association with patient satisfaction during a visit. Instead, the quality of the care provided was indicated in women's perception of time spent during the visit, which the authors suggest might depend on several qualitative factors for observation. Medical students' observations of provider-patient encounters and the use of narrative medicine have demonstrated positive learning outcomes for future providers. Student participation in documenting patient history (as demonstrated in the McDermott et al. 2019, study above) might also survey patient satisfaction and convey this valuable information as an assessment of clinical care given the time constraints for care in the clinical environment.

Ferrari et al. [15] conducted a qualitative study of women's perceptions of provider advice about diet and physical activity during pregnancy and found that women commonly reported overwhelming and confusing diet advice and paucity of physical activity advice that was limited to walking. The study involved a series of 13 focus groups with a total of 58 pregnant African American, Caucasian, and Hispanic women of varying body sizes [15]. Many women reported following the advice. However, when the advice was not followed, it was because women disagreed with it or simply did not want to do it. These findings suggest that even in reproductive medicine, women would benefit from more clear guidance from physicians and other providers regarding dietary choices and physical activity in pregnancy, and follow-up with patients to learn more about non-compliance with advice. With more information about their patients' lives and social behavior embedded within roles in families, providers can adapt dietary and physical activity advice in pregnancy to be both clear and individualized. Provider training should incorporate information gathering in follow-up appointments, and methods for offering and adapting such guidance multiple times throughout pregnancy, for example.

The literature supports an understanding of women's perceptions of providers as significant in determining their satisfaction with the experience, based on how expectations were or were not met [12] or time spent with the patient [13]. Patients' perceptions of providers also matter in the ways that mediate health outcomes such as compliance with medical advice perceived to be unclear or unfeasible within their social roles or lifestyles [15], and in the case of substance abuse, relatively unavailable from healthcare providers, despite receiving ample support from other programs and family support systems [11]. Medical providers who offer adequate attention to how women experience medical encounters, perceive expectations, understand guidance, form trust, and adopt recommendations for their health behavior can improve women's health outcomes and reduce health disparities. Doing so in any role, whether physicians or nurse practitioners, specialty-trained or general, or medical students, healthcare provides accomplish one of the IOM's most important competencies: patient-centered care.

Bias in Women's Treatment

Research indicates that bias against women shows up significantly in their health-care and treatment. There is overwhelming evidence that women's issues have been "ignored in patriarchal systems" [16]. Characterized as the "Yentl Syndrome," women are more likely to be treated less aggressively in their initial encounters with the healthcare system until they prove they are as sick as male patients present or are assumed to be. Heath [16] identified numerous areas in which this inequity shows up. Examples include:

(a) Drugs—women react differently to medication than men, yet most studies are conducted with male populations.
(b) Alcohol—women metabolize alcohol differently than men.
(c) Heart Disease—leading cause of death for both men and women, yet all studies are done on male subjects.
(d) Hypoglycemia—women on average normally have lower blood sugar level.
(e) Research problems—women have never been adequately represented in health research.
(f) Professional attitudes—the medical community continues to mishandle women's health concerns through negligence, sexism, and sheer inertia.

These differences have a significant impact on women's health resulting in differing needs in health, treatment, and medication.

Services for Women

Haseltine's [17] book *Our Bodies, Ourselves* set a precedence in offering guidance and encouragement to women to help them "learn about themselves and demystify their obstetric and gynecologic care." The book is groundbreaking in giving women access to information so that they could become informed not only about tests and procedures and bodily health, but they could be encouraged to become better health agents that ask questions to more actively participate in their own care. Women are the primary consumers of general healthcare services, including mental health [18]. As such, they consume services for themselves and serve as gatekeepers for others. Women often negotiate, mediate, and seek services on behalf of children, partners, parents, and other family members [19]. Women also serve as unpaid caregivers to family members providing essential support for private healthcare [18, 19]. A 2012 NPR health poll [20] found that 78% of women 40 years or older were aware of guidelines and when they should start regular mammograms compared to 67% of men 50 or older and their awareness of similar guidelines for prostate cancer screening [20]. Hucko [21] suggests that market sensitivity to women as consumers, using female-friendly messages in health campaigns targeted toward women, might be an effective strategy to expand health outreach [21]. Because women are primary consumers of healthcare, they carry a burden to understand the constant changes in the healthcare system. Unfortunately, health knowledge and awareness do not always translate into health behavior or self-advocacy.

Bertakis et al. [9] examined gender differences in the utilization of healthcare services. In this study, new adult patients ($N = 509$) were randomly assigned to primary care physicians at a university medical center. Their use of healthcare services and associated charges were monitored for 1 year of care. A self-reported health status was measured using the Medical Outcomes Study Short Form (see [9] for more information), indicating that women had significantly lower self-reported health status and lower mean education. Juxtaposed with research about service provision, women's (under) utilization of services is less clear. For example, Terplan [22] obtained characteristics of facilities from the National Survey of Substance Abuse Treatment Services and treatment need data from the National Survey on Drug Use and Health. He examined differences in the provision of women-centered programs by urbanization level in data from the National Center for Health Statistics 2006 Rural-Urban County Continuum. The results of the study indicated that of the 13,000 facilities surveyed annually, the proportion offering women-centered services significantly declined from 43% in 2002 to 40% in 2009 ($P < 0.001$). Urban location, state population size, and Medicaid payments predicted the provision of such services as trauma-related and domestic violence counseling, child care, and housing assistance (all, $P < 0.001$). The prevalence of women with unmet needs ranged from 81% to 95% across states. A major conclusion of the study was that the change in availability of women-centered drug treatment services was minimal from 2002 to 2009, even though the need for treatment was high in all states. The research suggests that characteristics of geographic location and economic circumstances may be correlated with women's underutilization of services, despite their availability.

According to Stolp and Fox [23], "[b]aseline assessments [of service provision] indicate there is much room for improvement in receipt of preventive services among women" [23]. The preventive services coverage requirement and other provisions of the ACA have increased access to preventive care and optimized the opportunity for women to receive recommended clinical preventive services. Stolp and Fox's [23] study suggests that if these opportunities are fully realized and leveraged, the increasing use of preventive services could allow more American women to enjoy longer, healthier lives from the timely detection and response to preventable adverse health conditions [23].

A Pilot Study of Practitioner Perceptions of Women's Experiences in Medicine

Medical sociologists describe a curious contradiction in medicalization and health research during the 1970s, 80s, and 90s, which may be relevant here: while the process of medicalization restricted its scope to women, and social science research excluded studies of men's experiences, men's bodies remained normative in clinical and epidemiological research on diseases, such as heart disease and cancer [2]. This trend reversed during pertinent biomedical transformations in medical practice to focus on the medicalization of masculinities and enhancement of the male body, for example. Biomedicalization shifted the use of technologies from problematizing women's health to explorations of the male body's functioning as indicative of the "natural" body, ranging from research on hormonal influences on behavior and ability, to sexual performance and reproduction, to chemical neurology in handling everyday stress. For example, life situations for women in modern society are complicated, often as the "Dr. Mom" role can take a toll on women or other role conflicts (as economic providers and caretakers in multiple family situations) create strain on women's health and ability to manage their own health.

Clarke et al. [2] suggest that in all areas of medical advancement and research—even in developing cellular knowledge about the human body—we are encouraged to ask and answer the question of generalizability to women, just as we have had to do so for decades. "Natural" for whom? While women's bodies (and health) have been historically problematized in medicine, and society for that matter, advancements in medical knowledge and technology continue to perpetuate a social hierarchy with men situated as the explicit focus for care, and women as subordinates, with limited agency and power to change the medical structures that treat them [2].

The present pilot study aims to test the feasibility (and relevance) of qualitative research in further understanding women's treatment in health, prior to undertaking a larger study that would potentially use mixed methods for investigation. We hope to highlight an association between provider's perceptions of women's treatment in healthcare and themes found in the current literature on women's health. We hope to offer suggestions for continuing action research in medical fields that underscores the medical education reform suggested above by McDermott, et al., 2019, which also supports the deployment of interdisciplinary coordination across fields, and coordination of all ranks of professionals, in the service of patient-centered, quality care.[1]

Lahane Thabane et al. [24] state that "the rationale for a pilot study can be grouped under several broad classifications," "the main goal of … [which] is to

---

[1] The present study underwent Expedited Review by the Protection of Human Subjects Committee (PHSC) at the College of William and Mary in Williamsburg, VA and was approved in April 2018. Questions about the conceptual design and methodology of this work may be directed to either of the authors, while questions about ethics may be directed to Dr. Jennifer Stevens, Chair of PHSC, William & Mary, at jastev@wm.edu

assess feasibility" [24–26]. In the case of the present pilot study, researchers conducted the survey without funding, independent from full-time academic roles which are not unrelated to medical research and the work of practitioners but are also not exclusively focused on either aspect of the fields addressed herein. Neither researcher possessed nor gained privileged access to population datasets on women's health other than that which was publicly available or represented in the literature. Time and resource restrictions, in part, limited the research process to feasible means of the study below: a qualitative survey and the use of Geographic Information Systems (GIS) mapping to speculate continuing scholarship.

Methods

Researchers used purposive sampling to identify a variety of practitioners in the field of medicine and invited them to answer open-ended questions in a questionnaire about their roles as practitioners, training for their most current position(s), years of experience in the field, and perceptions about women's treatment in healthcare based on their encounters in medical settings. (The Providers' Perceptions of Women's Experiences questionnaire is included in Appendix B, with researchers' envelope communication with participants and consent statement.) While limitations of this approach might include the possibility of bias on the part of researchers, wherein the sampling neglects to identify a comprehensive or representative range of respondents to contribute an empirically generalizable understanding of the phenomenon being studied, generalizability is not the intended outcome nor value of a pilot study [24, 27].

The survey and consent form were e-mailed in 2018 to 29 healthcare practitioners identified in a purposive sample of medical professionals across fields and position types. Two follow-up e-mails were sent to yield a total of nine ($N = 9$) completed surveys. The areas of healthcare practice of professionals varied. Areas of focus and specialty represented a wide range, nonetheless: family medicine, dentistry, pharmacy, emergency nursing, corporate healthcare, health sciences, and pediatrics. (Two of the practitioners have since transitioned into administrative roles.) Over half of the respondents had more than 10 years of experience as healthcare professionals.

Results

Respondents overwhelmingly agreed that women's experiences were different from men in hospital and clinical settings, but thought they might not be different in other medical settings. Some described differences in how providers were perceived, while others focused on women's treatment. Related to perceptions of providers, responses indicate that the gendered nature of medical encounters is a mutual dynamic:

> [W]omen are not recognized as providers [in the clinical setting]. Patients usually assume you are the nurse…. Also, respect is not automatic as a female.

Another noted that patients seemed to show a different "level of comfort with a different sex of the provider, particularly in nursing," a field occupied by women. Blau and Kahn's [28] study of gender gaps in educational and occupational attainment shows "a dramatic shift in the occupational choices of women in the US, with the female share of graduates in law, medical, and business schools rising by a factor of five [in the last four decades]" (in [28, 29]). If responses in our study can be replicated on a larger scale, it would be interesting to explore the impact of greater female representation in provider roles, on medical boards, and on health policy on both men and women's experiences in treatment. When asked what could be done about these interactions, a respondent suggested "more patients and healthcare workers having experience with a diverse set of providers" and in particular, "allow men to become more comfortable (we assume, as patients) in clinical settings."

Providers also observed: "Women tend to ask more questions and research conditions. Men are not always as forthcoming." One respondent cited medicine's traditional focus on "[m]ale biology [as] the default mode in the history of research in medicine, with the exception of obstetrics and gynecology" in describing observations of women's undertreatment as compared to men:

> There are standard doses of medications and since…it is absorbed/metabolized at different rates it could lead to women's pain being undertreated or receiving too much of a pain medication which could lead to other health problems.

The same respondent gave an example about differences in the way that men and women express symptoms of a heart attack, noting that women "are more likely to present with sweating and pain in their back or other symptoms that are not always associated with a heart attack" such as the better-known "classic symptoms [of] chest pain/tightness over the heart and trouble breathing—something almost every male having a heart attack presents with." They add:

> While I have not witnessed any examples of women receiving poorer treatment than men due to blatant sexism, I believe that due to the way medicine was researched throughout history there is an unconscious bias that can lead to women being treated differently than men in healthcare settings.

This respondent also noted that with continuing reforms in medical training, "differences in physiognomy/anatomy are now more widely known" so treatment is improving with knowledge of differences in men and women's symptomology for the same disease process. They believed that "[c]ontinuing community outreach and empowering people to take control of their healthcare will cause the biggest changes."

Almost all respondents answered "Definitely Yes" to having observed a correlation between women living in poverty, or low-income neighborhoods, with their likelihood of developing chronic illnesses such as heart disease, diabetes, or hypertension (and others) across all racial groupings. (The remaining response was "Probably Yes.") Asked how they could assess the income or educational level of patients; they specified several approaches:

- *Health Literacy and Comprehension:* "I am able to identify it in the way they describe their symptoms and, in their ability, to understand the information given by a provider."
- *Direct Communication:* "ask about where they live, job, insurance status."
- *Interpretive Observation:* "[Their] grammar and engagement in their care."

One respondent elaborated on the system and process of care as being problematic:

> The biggest part is follow-up care. I work in a non-profit hospital, so we provide financial assistance/charity care and a lot of patients have told me that they come to the Emergency Department because their PCP won't see them. While we can see and treat their current symptoms in the Emergency [Department], we cannot follow their healthcare the way that a primary physician could.

This respondent noted that they often saw the same patients returning for the same symptoms "because their chronic health problems are not well managed."

Our respondents' observations of the impact of economic limitations on patients' experiences also reveal factors beyond their immediate control as care providers, with the most frequent attention paid to the (in)affordability of medication and some attention to what could be characterized as cascading effects in other areas of health including lack of access to healthy foods, lack of access to transportation for medical care, dental care, inability to afford medical tests such as labs and imaging exams, inability to afford the cost of physician's visits, inability to exercise choice in medications, and (un)timeliness of specialty appointments.

Regarding racism and discrimination in treatment, almost all respondents answered that they had "Definitely" or "Probably Yes" witnessed racial bias and treatment. One respondent observed: "Physicians sometimes assume that African American are less informed and concerned about their health." Several respondents indicated that this provider's perception often resulted in conducting a limited history with the patient, offering fewer diagnostic choices, spending less time with patients, or assumptions about drug-seeking behavior that delimited pain management and medication. In response to a question about what could be done about racial bias in treatment, one resigned participant answered "not much" while another suggested professional training on unconscious bias in treatment. An optimistic response in the study relied on the dynamics of the team for reform:

> The good thing is that where I work, we are a team of people, with attending physicians, residents, nurses, EMTs, and nurse techs. It helps to hold each other accountable and follow-up on patient complaints/concerns. If a patient appears in pain and pain control is not initially ordered, the nurse, tech, etc., will address that with the provider.

The range of responses from more resigned to more proactive and based on an interdisciplinary team approach could indicate the variation in training amid our respondents (by field and position), or even medical education transitions over the course of a career. Certainly, the last response demonstrates the feasibility of change in contexts of units' interactions as professionals with one another as well as with patients.

Respondents suggested that women's life circumstances frequently complicated their quality of care in the following ways, primarily due to the role strain on women as mothers and as working caretakers "who may have to take off to care for children or elderly parents."

> I often hear women say that they have felt poorly for some time, but they were taking care of their elderly parents, take care of their kids, working, etc. I hear "excuses" from women as to why they put their healthcare off fairly often and I do not hear this often from men.

Respondents additionally shared their views on whether disparities existed for women in areas of Funding for Research, Specialized Clinical Settings, and Health Policies. Specifically, they were asked "With regard to issues that are specific to women's healthcare (e.g., breast cancer and screening or prevention measures, sexual and reproduction health, maternity care, etc.), do you feel women's healthcare also reveals disparities in the following settings?" [See Table 3.1 for the distribution of answers in all categories.]

Women, regardless of education or income level, are most likely to be primary caretakers within their family systems—as wives, mothers, and daughters of aging relatives [30]. As a result, women face a gauntlet of decisions, institutions, and challenges to access healthcare [30]. In Chen et al.'s [31] critique of the Family Medical Leave Act, researchers call attention to the high burden of caregiving as a social need in our aging population. Women, Hispanic employees, and low-wage workers (who predominantly occupy temporary, part-time, or short-term worker positions) are not likely to be paid sick and family leave when caring for elderly family members, because the policy does not extend to all employees. Benefits of paid leave are limited to defined circumstances of "serious health" in which caretaking needs and informal roles that women play are not easily, or formally documented for review and approval [31].

The present study suggests that in a larger study we might expect to find: (1) differential behavior of men and women as patients in the clinical setting, with men repressing communication in contact with female providers and women asking more questions, and (2) differential life circumstances as competing factors for individual healthcare, compliance with prescribed health behavior and managing appointments, especially in contexts of family care systems.

Table 3.1 Distribution of answers—providers' perceptions of women's experiences

	Definitely yes	Probably yes	Might or might not	Probably not
Funding for research	3	3	4	1
Specialized clinical settings	3	3	2	0
Health policies	2	3	2	0

Note. Providers' Perceptions of Women's Experiences

Discussion

What do healthcare providers learn from encounters with women as patients in their clinical settings? To answer this question, the authors conducted a literature review for themes in women's healthcare outcomes as well as in encounters with healthcare providers. Then, based on themes in the literature we conducted a pilot survey of medical professionals to gather initial reports on what they had observed in varied capacities of care. Importantly, the authors' focus on women as patients does not intend to frame a women's experience as merely passive recipients of care. Instead, we aim to shed light on the multiple circumstances and roles at play in the clinical encounter, a situation in which medical staff at all levels can learn from the women they treat how best to care for them. Outside medical clinics, women live as individuals who are also spouses, daughters, caregivers, mothers, and so on. Women's attention to health occurs within the more powerful social dynamics of family and their occupational contexts. The medical encounter is undeniably an important opportunity for healthcare providers to engage their patients responsively and effectively, but their engagement with health need not be limited to assessment and treatment activities, performed in abstraction from the contexts of human interaction that occur in clinical settings and broader health systems.

First, practitioners commented on patient reactions to female providers in their fields, or in their areas of practice, sometimes connecting the lack of diversity in their field to the comfort level of patients who must seek care from a different sex. Occupational change takes time, but continued gender tension (due to unfamiliarity with female providers on the part of men) is represented by the responses. This pilot study joins other research supporting scholarship and recruitment efforts to attract women to STEM fields, and included in this, medicine at all levels of practice and authority. Two respondents noted specifically the historical orientation to the male body in research and suggested also that research bias toward men impacted women's treatment in healthcare settings, whether they observed blatant interpersonal sexism or not. The distribution of their responses to questions about research funding, clinical settings, and health policies leans toward the latter two areas of research. Our study suggests that medical encounters and the policies that determine a process for treatment remain most salient for understanding women's treatment in medicine, as perceived by providers.

Second, most practitioners confirmed findings in the literature—that women who live in poverty (or low-income household or neighborhoods) are disproportionately more likely to develop heart disease, diabetes, hypertension, and other major illnesses across racial groupings.

They were able to identify the income or educational level of women patients by taking cues from their conversation. Practitioners made assessments based on a patient's grammar, the way they describe their symptoms, and their ability to understand the information given by a provider. The type of insurance coverage or lack of insurance also provided cues for the practitioners. Practitioners observed the impact of limited economic resources on their overall experience with healthcare and their ability to manage an illness. Health outcomes manifested through several social circumstances, including access to healthy foods, ability to purchase medication and medical tests, and failure to comply with treatment plans. The lack of access to transportation led to missed visits and inability to follow up on treatment. Our study suggests that a systems approach to medical care might lead to more effective management of chronic illnesses and improve health outcomes in targeted regions, based on economic and population analyses.

Third, our research suggests that the social experience of racism and discrimination carries over into the clinical experiences of women as patients. Many respondents indicated that they have or probably witnessed what they consider racial bias. One respondent indicated that "respect is not automatic as a female." Practitioners have witnessed this bias by observing providers who lower expectations for what the patient can do, and who may not push them enough to make diagnosis considerations. In addition, physicians sometimes assume that African Americans are less informed and concerned about their health. Practitioners also observed physicians making assumptions based on appearance without even asking and doing proper history. Also, they observed physicians not sharing all potential treatment options given assumption that person cannot pay, and assuming African American patients are drug-seeking during acute pain crisis. While many trainings on bias and confronting differences in medicine exist, we recommend those that align closely with the organizational and medical priorities set by the IOM and others—those that emphasize competencies in the following areas: (1) to provide patient-centered care, (2) to work in interdisciplinary teams, (3) to employ evidence-based practice, (4) to apply quality improvement, and (5) to utilize informatics [3]. (See the still relevant work of Tervalon, M. and Murray-García, J [32] on cultural humility versus cultural competence approaches in physician training; the content is also available in a creative presentation on YouTube, see https://youtu.be/SaSHLbS1V4w).

Implications for Future Research: Two Kinds of Mapping

Current medical practice and treatment emphasize technoscientific advancements in diagnosis, treatment, and in preventing genetic as well as cellular disease. Advancements in the precision with which technological and scientific tools can diagnose and treat the human body also lead to assumptions of greater manipulability in health and knowledge about human health. Greater manipulability has been historically problematic for women despite whatever benefits advanced knowledge yielded—for example, in cases of body enhancement surgeries that result in infection, compounded illness, or even death. Also, biomedical approaches to health profoundly influence behavioral dynamics between individuals by dictating how health information is communicated, in determining which factors to prioritize for research funding and advancement, in prioritizing scientific data above other indicators of the human body, and in shaping cultural expectations for both health maintenance and delivery, for example [5]. Building theoretically on our pilot study, our ideas for future study integrate two disciplinary areas with medical research: (1) big data analysis as part of coordinating clinical training, treatment, and information management between organizations in a region and (2) the use of and family systems mapping in managing follow-up for patient-centered care that is embedded in social contexts.

Big Data analysis warrants attention at all levels and settings of medical treatment within an increasingly complex biomedical industry of healthcare in the US. "Big Data" refers to "extremely large data sets that may be analyzed computationally to reveal patterns, trends, and associations, especially relating to human behavior and interactions" (Oxford Languages Dictionary, 2020). The unfortunate circumstance of COVID-19 has made evident the usefulness of large data analysis in communicating and analyzing cases and rates of infection, broken down geographic location in varying regions, such as state and county. A prominent example is the publicly available mapping site managed by the Johns Hopkins University's Coronavirus Resource Center, demonstrating tracking, critical trends analyses, US and global maps, and even tracking across time (see https://coronavirus.jhu.edu/us-map). At the writing of this chapter, this map is one among many across states, counties, and districts being used across disciplines in health fields, natural, and social sciences to project and imagine human health outcomes over time. Population, health, and changes in health are better understood in the dynamic ways that they realistically occur. GIS mapping presents a way to see community change (including economic and social variables of change) using larger datasets to illuminate actual, versus abstract contexts for managing local healthcare. What follows is a broad overview of US demographics and women's health, as context for considering future research directions.

From 2014 to 2018, the United States had a total population of 322.9 million—163.9 million (50.8%) females and 159.0 million (49.2%) males. The median age was 37.9 years. An estimated 22.8% of the population was under 18 years, 36.0% was 18 to 44 years, 26.0% was 45–64 years, and 15.2% was 65 years and older. For people reporting one race alone, 72.7% were White; 12.7% were Black or African American; 0.8% were American Indian; Alaska Native; 5.4% were Asian; 0.2% were Native Hawaiian and Other Pacific Islander, and 4.9% were some other race. An estimated 3.2% reported two or more races. An estimated 17.8% of the people in the United States were Hispanic. An estimated 61.1% of the people in the United States were White non-Hispanic. (American Community Survey (ACS), www.2020census.gov). By 2050, non-Hispanic White females are projected to no longer be the majority (46.1%) and about one-third of females will be Hispanic (29.9%) [33]. It is not entirely clear how that projection will translate in terms of healthcare needs and treatment, except to anticipate greater culturally and linguistically appropriate health services. Women's Health USA (2012, [33]) reported that more than one in five Hispanic (29.5%), non-Hispanic [sic] Black (23.2%), Native Hawaiian/Pacific Islander (20.8%) women reported poor health, as compared to about 13% of White and non-Hispanic Asian women. Non-Hispanic black, Hispanic, and non-Hispanic American Indian/Alaska Native women are "disproportionately affected by several diseases and adverse health conditions, including diabetes, high blood pressure, overweight and obesity, asthma, HIV/AIDS, and sexually transmitted infections" [33].

The agency of Healthcare Research and Quality indicates that health insurance facilitates entry into the healthcare system. Uninsured people are less likely to receive medical care, and more likely to be in poor health status (https://www.ahrq.gov). Among the civilian noninstitutionalized population in the United States in 2014–2018, 90.6% had health insurance coverage and 9.4% did not have health insurance coverage. Private coverage was 67.7% and government coverage was 34.7%, respectively. The percentage of children under the age of 19 with no health insurance coverage was 5.2% (https://www.census.gov/acs/www/data/data-tables-and-tools/narrative-profiles/2018/reports). According to the National Health Interview Survey Early Release Program, in 2019, 33.2 million (10.3%) persons of all ages were uninsured at the time of the interview. Hispanic adults (29.7%) were more likely than non-Hispanic black (14.7%), non-Hispanic white (10.5%) and non-Hispanic Asian (7.5%) to be uninsured. Although men (16.3%) were more likely than women to be uninsured, among adults age 18–64, women were more likely to experience delayed or non-receipt of care (National Health Interview Survey Early Release Program, 2019; National Center for Health Statistics, 2018). See Table 3.2 for more information.

The Agency for Healthcare Research and Quality emphasizes that the lack of timeliness can result in emotional distress, physical harm, and higher treatment costs. Timely delivery of appropriate care can help reduce mortality and morbidity for chronic conditions. This report also indicated that from 2005–2012, females were significantly more likely than males to be delayed or unable to get needed medical care, dental care, or prescription medicines in the past 12 months, as observed by providers in our pilot study. See Table 3.3 for more information.

Table 3.2 Experience of delayed or non-receipt of care by gender 2017

	Delay or non-receipt of needed medical care due to cost, 2017	Non-receipt of needed prescription drugs due to cost, 2017	Non-receipt of needed dental care due to cost
Male	9.1%	5.0%	9.3%
Female	10.8%	8.0%	13.7%

Note. National Health Interview Survey Early Release Program, 2019; National Center for Health Statistics, 2018

Table 3.3 Experience of delayed or non-receipt of care 2005–2012

Delay or unable to get medical care, dental care, medicines		
	2005	2012
Male	9.9%	9.4%
Female	12.8%	11.6%

Note. Agency for Healthcare Research and Quality

Sung et al. [34] suggest that health disparities for women have a structural basis for inequity in communities. Sung et al. [34] combine data from the 2001–2012 editions of the US Behavioral Risk Factor Surveillance System (BRFSS) with annual regional inequality measures to construct an individual-level data set that will "incorporate potential lagged effects of income inequality and vary the geographic scope of... analysis between states (higher level of geography) and counties (lower level of geography)" in assessing the variance in findings across geographic communities. Using seven measures of health outcomes, Sung et al. [34] found statistically significant evidence supporting the income inequality hypothesis (IIH) which is "the notion that everyone's health in society is reduced with more income inequality" and the relative deprivation hypothesis (RDH) which "suggests that health status is influenced by how one's income compares to others." Researchers also found statistically significant evidence that both income inequality and relative deprivation evidence that both income inequality and relative deprivation lead to reductions in exercise and access to care; and, that relative deprivation also statistically significantly increases smoking and drinking [34].

The economic mismatch between women living in poverty with contemporary markets for distributing and managing healthcare, as situated within geographies of inequality, and embedded in experiences of poverty, is especially alarming when considering the rising cost of treatments due to market changes. Diversified healthcare distribution furthermore translates into multiple sites to visit in the health marketplace, with varied, and complicated options for Medicaid or subsidized healthcare (for the uninsured), or multiple co-payments (for the insured) [5]. Time and money expenditures can become barriers for the working class or lower income women whose job and family obligations and income budgets do not accommodate irregular visits to a doctor's office.

Many healthcare facilities additionally require patients to interface with staff and doctors via e-technologies for scheduling appointments, acquiring updates on tests and screenings, and even communicating with the doctor in some cases. Such practices establish a false equivalency among individuals in assuming shared responsibility for health maintenance via electronic health information recordkeeping and presumes access to the Internet as a source of information. (COVID-19 has revealed the benefit of technology on its own terms for sustaining healthcare services, but we are already seeing differential health outcomes among those with limited access to care in all its forms, a continuing problem in healthcare delivery.) Obtaining information about healthcare via medical websites is not (on its own) a reliable source for adequate healthcare information (retrieval and management) and decision-making. The use of medical websites without critical health literacy can lead to dangerous self-treatment, errors in understanding illness, and delays in consulting a medical professional [5].

A Model for GIS Healthcare Analysis

Terplan's [22] study demonstrated that urban location, state population size, and Medicaid payments predicted the provision of women-centered services (such as trauma-related and domestic violence counseling, childcare, and housing assistance), while women's needs were largely unmet due to underutilization. The present authors assert that the social circumstances themselves determine the observed outcome of underutilization and therefore warrant further investigation and assertive response by the medical community. While not all the circumstances mentioned are embedded solely in poor communities, the likelihood of their occurrence compounded with a lack of access is high among the poor. Below we present a case in which GIS analyses might be engaged (by medical students, research collaborators, etc.) based on measures of social vulnerability and women's health outcomes in varied regions.

Methodology

The following maps were created in ArcGIS Pro 2.6. Using data from the Centers for Disease Control and Prevention, tabular data was converted into shapefiles for mapping purposes. Maps were curated by manipulating symbology to reflect the variables of interest. Statistical analysis was not performed; however, some spatial trends are suggested. Further statistical and spatial analysis is needed to reveal any associations between variables. Using this methodology, more maps could be created based on different health measures such as heart disease or diabetes or social measures.[2] The maps in Fig. 3.1 represent aggregate level data drawn from the CDC [35] Social Vulnerability Index database and from the US Cancer Statistics Data Visualizations Tool [36] developed by the US Cancer Statistics Working Group. The Social Vulnerability Index (SVI) includes the following variables to assess the social vulnerability of a community: Socioeconomic Status, Household Composition and Disability, Minority Status and Language, and Housing Type and Transportation (see [36], for more sub-categorical information). Figure 3.2 represents aggregate data on Female Cancer Mortality, but other variables such as disease prevalence are also available.

The authors selected Virginia and Iowa as state region case studies that geographically contextualize several of our pilot study respondents' practices. The Agency for Healthcare Research and Quality [6] suggested that mid-United States regions, urban as well as rural locations, and low-income areas should be prioritized in designing and delivering patient-centered care. The CDC data used to create the following maps is represented at the county level of analysis, and both states contain counties that might be characterized in the variety of ways recommended for redress.

---

[2] Many thanks to Olivia Spencer, GIS Fellow in the Center for Geospatial Analysis at William and Mary, for her authorship in creating the maps and insight for considering comparative cases.

Social Vulnerability Index in Virginia by County

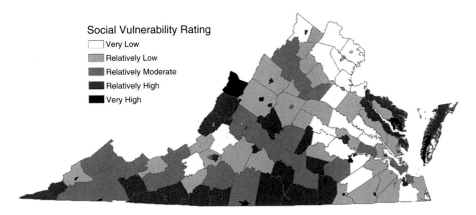

Fig. 3.1 Virginia, US map: social vulnerability index by county

Female Cancer Mortality in Virginia by County

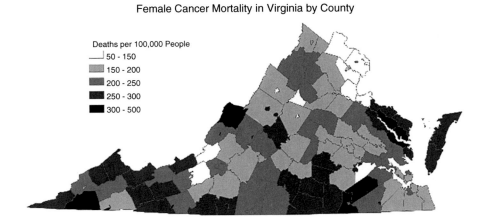

Fig. 3.2 Virginia, US map: female cancer mortality by county

Preliminary Analyses

In this section, we offer a brief analysis of the data as presented for Virginia (VA) and Iowa (IA), regarding measures of the social vulnerability index and the prevalence of cancer mortality among women. In Virginia, the following counties indicated the highest levels of social vulnerability (see Fig. 3.1): Emporia City, Norton City, Galax City, Petersburg City, and Martinsville City. The counties in Virginia with the highest levels of female cancer mortality among women (also, see Fig. 3.2) include Dickenson County, Buena Vista City, Lunenburg County, Tazewell County, and Mecklenburg County. There are no overlaps in these lists, but visual overlap is identifiable in Nelson County, at the Relatively High Level for SVI and a Relatively High Level for Female Cancer Mortality. Nelson County might be characterized as a mixed rural and suburban part of Charlottesville, VA, itself surrounded by other similarly rural/suburban counties that include mountains and waterways.

Further region-based analysis might consider patients' proximity or access to the University of Virginia Medical Center for diagnosis and treatment for female cancer, evaluating the negative or positive impact of proximity and access (e.g., screening, transportation) on disease prevalence monitoring and reporting.

Researchers may add another feature layer for this map to indicate cancer treatment centers in the region and coordinate care according to a variety of other social determinants. For example, counties located on the interior and outer peninsulas of the state show higher levels of female cancer mortality, suggesting there may be an environmental impact of water quality on women's health in the state. The Tye River, which flows through Nelson County, is by way of the James River a watershed of the Chesapeake Bay. Certainly, there may be many explanations, such as the existence (or history) of harmful agriculture (e.g., tobacco industry), commercial production (e.g., coal-fired power plants), but with added data analysis preventive care and health education might directly address health outcomes such as cancer in women with region-specific advisories or campaigns. Lastly, counties at the southern border of Virginia indicate the borderless character of human health, wherein recognition of human beings' regional coexistence, movement, and the necessity for health coordination is made visual. Interdependence for healthcare management and coordination, especially for federal resources, might be facilitated by interstate communication and efforts which contextualize the work of clinics, hospitals, and practices of all kinds within the region.

Iowa presents an interesting comparison case. In Iowa, counties with higher levels of SVI (see Fig. 3.3) include Ringgold County, Montgomery County, Wayne

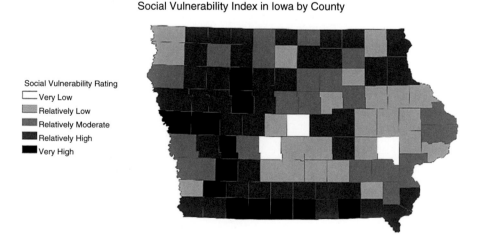

Fig. 3.3 Iowa, US Map: social vulnerability index by county

County, Decatur County, and Pocahontas County. Counties with a higher prevalence of Female Cancer Mortality (also, see Fig. 3.4) include Emmet county,
Ringgold County, Calhoun County, Guthrie County, and Monroe county.

Similar to the Iowa case it is easier to identify the possibility of a correlation
between SVI and Female Cancer Mortality as indicated by the presence of Ringgold
County, IA in each map; but statistical analysis of multiple factors would give
researchers a better understanding of the significance of those factors.

The public availability of data opens the possibility of statistical analyses that
include other geographically located determinants of health, such as the availability
of specialized treatment and care centers, agricultural and manufacturing exposure
to contaminants that lead to cancer in specified health districts or county regions.
(Notably, the southern border and southwestern tip of Iowa demonstrate once again
the likelihood of shared health experiences among patients in neighboring states
Kentucky and Tennessee, which contain rural Appalachian communities, mountains, and waterways that might impact health significantly in terms of access,
despite each state's having urban centers.) County-specific data enables healthcare
officials to target disease management of many kinds of regions, in correspondence
with the state distribution of resources for prioritized healthcare. Our maps represent static maps that selected Female Cancer Mortality prevalence. But other measures of disease prevalence are available and can generate inquiries about other
chronic diseases such as diabetes and heart disease. Static maps help to visualize
geographic patterns in a succinct manner. Spatial patterns that might not be obvious
in a large data set can be more easily revealed in static maps. Interactive maps on the
other hand allow for collaboration between researchers and the inclusion of spatial
data at various scales to promote data-driven information that is digestible to medical practitioners.

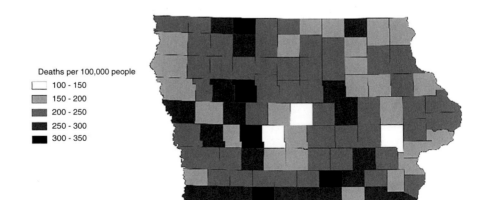

Fig. 3.4 Iowa, US map: female cancer mortality by county

Family Mapping in Healthcare Assessment

Bowen Theory offers researchers, educators, consultants, and practitioners across disciplines a framework for assessing and tracking human functioning as embedded in multigenerational contexts of family systems (Bowen, 1978; Keller & Noone, 2020).

> When combined with research methods, a Bowen theory systems orientation for family research includes: (1) observation—the primary task of the systems oriented researcher and the core element of science; (2) facts—observable behavior that can be objectively and scientifically established; and (3) family diagram—an assessment procedure designed to collect observable and factual data that provide a multigenerational diagrammatic description of the relationships and emotional patterns within the nuclear and extended family system; and (4) behavioral markers—observable and factual data that are indicators of the emotional process in the family relationship system….).[3]

Victoria Harrison (2018), Director of the Center for the Study of Natural Systems and the Family in Houston, Texas, developed a guide for using family diagramming as a method for mapping human health, which is the focus of this section. Family diagramming is a method for mapping the situated facts of functioning for individuals within the larger contexts of their families. In addition to documenting family relationships (including caretaking roles), diagrams can also document birth, deaths, marriages, divorces, migration and geographical moves, education, military service, criminal history, health history, social symptoms (such as alcohol or drug use), fertility and reproduction, and other stressful life events that impact human health and health behavior (Harrison, 2018). To the extent possible, Harrison models the work of Holmes and Rahe (1967) Life Events Stress Scale (studied extensively by other MDs and health researcher in the 40 years since its development) to map family systems iteratively, alongside biofeedback in coaching clients, particularly around the areas of infertility and reproduction. She states that by using precise information about existing and past generations (to the extent possible) "[o]ne can begin to consider more factually the challenges present around the time of birth, an affair, marriage or separation, or the onset of symptoms and diagnoses."

The following family maps are fictitious case representations of how Bowen Theory facilitates methods of observation, documenting facts, diagramming family relationships, and accounting for behavioral markers as they present in clinical settings and relate to health outcomes. (See Jamison, 2014 and Charon, et al., 2017 for compelling uses of case study and narrative medicine to illustrate and illuminate medical practice and methodologies for examining modes of intervention toward improvement.) They offer intentionally structured differences between family

---

[3] See Bowen (1978) or Keller and Noone (2020) for an in-depth overview of the theory, used in fields ranging from psychology to medicine to organizational consultation world-wide.

circumstances in which women might rely on partners or not, to share resources and experience relative stability due to educational credentials, financial resources, or extended family relationships. Of course, no family structure guarantees stability, making the case for particularized assessments even more important. In order to illustrate the potential usefulness of family diagramming, family structure differences are distinguished purposely below.

Case #1: Meredith

Meredith (see Fig. 3.5) is a 50-year-old professional woman with an advanced degree, presenting with chronic back pain that results in visits to the Emergency Department. She is a married mother of three, all under the age of 18, and designated caretaker for her mother recently relocated to an assisted living community. Meredith's pain is located primarily in her lower back and shoulders. With good health insurance, she has had a series of imaging tests that show slight arthritis and degenerative disc disease within "normal" range for her age. Her blood pressure is slightly elevated in ED visits and differs from measures in clinical visits which she undergoes routinely for preventive care. In addition to a battery of health tests for assessing health, how might family diagramming inform ongoing care for this patient and family situation?

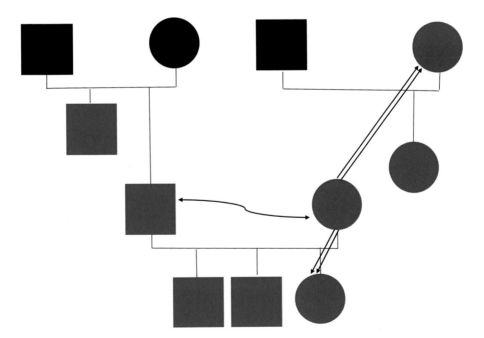

Fig. 3.5 Family diagram case #1: Meredith

Based on our literature review and on the responses from the pilot study, women's family and social circumstances routinely pose challenges to health and behaviors that would improve health. While providers recognize the impact of external circumstances on women's health, few have time or make time to assess and track those situations. The family diagram in Fig. 3.5 illustrates the situation in which a woman patient undergoes caregiving stressors (directed primarily at her mother in senior care and youngest child, her only daughter). Working as a full-time professional, she likely has little time for other responsibilities such as household maintenance, exercise, or tracking financial and health well-being on her own. Depending on her partner's share in assuming responsibilities (to extended family as well as this nuclear unit), stressors can vary (by availability of other adult siblings, health and status of parents, employment, and their own health status). The family diagram can serve as a clinical shortcut (by hand or using technology) for doctors, nurses, social workers, or medical students to document observations of the patient while intake assessment occurs, note facts about the patient in family contexts (such as age, health, and lifestyle routine), diagram relationships (as patients report them in terms of caregiving, conflict, cooperation, etc.), and assess the impact of behavioral factors on the patient's health. For example, if the patient above presents repeatedly with elevated pain and blood pressure, medical staff can also ask about relationships (such as last visit to the mother, having a good relationship with the partner, health of child, for example) to assess any correlation with flares in pain and patient's practical ability to maintain health. A professional woman who is also a mother and primary caregiver in her home may have little "bandwidth" for recommendations of rest or additional time allocation in physical therapy. Referrals to support services may be more effective, especially if prior recommendations have not adequately addressed the problem.

But what if Meredith were a single parent undergoing a period of unemployment with a high school education? Even a slight adjustment to family diagram above alters the kinds of questions and observations that a clinician might make. For an alternate map, see the case of Mandy below.

Case #2: Mandy
If the patient Mandy (see Fig. 3.6) presented with similar symptoms, we might see that even the slightest adjustment in circumstances related to family context can alter pressure on a person's resources, health, and behavioral patterns. Mandy may be less reliant on a partner for shared resources for financial well-being (and therefore shelter and food) or for caregiving responsibilities related to children, depending on the household composition, relationship status with children's father or other partners, and the characteristics of that relationship (cooperative, conflictual, voluntary, or legally mandated, for example). Likewise, Mandy may be dependent on older children for caregiving support (shifting relationship strain and stability according to differences in capabilities), and further stretched for financial resources and seeking healthcare without insurance coverage for herself or her children. She

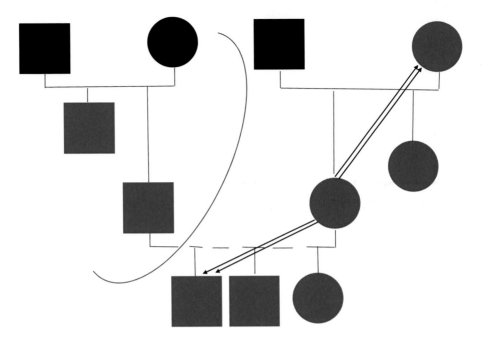

Fig. 3.6 Family diagram case #2: Mandy

may have limited resources or control over the quality of care her mother receives, based on what is affordable, transportation to the care site, and access to social or legal resources that support elder care in families.

Healthcare providers can neither manage nor exert influence over the range of variations patients might experience in life stressors, but medical students, social workers, and nurses at varying levels can track life stressors and changes in a patient's profile, adding qualitative information to patient-centered care. Admittedly, life stressors themselves do not "diagnose" patients more adequately. Instead, they are suggested here as indicators for more responsive clinical care, interaction with patients, a more holistic assessment of patient needs, and alternative methods for communicating with patients about their health. Integrated with traditional assessment tools for collecting data on patients, family diagramming offers another tool for mediating and documenting information about patients in family contexts. Uploaded as an image document the use of family diagramming could translate into better treatment across practices, especially as eHealth technologies allow for shared information across clinical, hospital, and other medical institutions for a given patient. Population data reports on broader disease prevalence and breaks down circumstances demographically for an overview of human health at aggregate levels of generality. Family diagramming poses an opportunity for collecting information that is patient-centered, involving the patients themselves in sharing experiences of health and illness as part of their everyday lives.

Conclusion

Our pilot research suggests that women's treatment in healthcare environments must account for several social factors as observed by providers:

1. Sex-based relational dynamics and representation in medical occupations as indicative of broader cultural dynamics that influence health communication in the clinical setting;
2. Routinely observed impact of economic inequality and a lack of resources (financial, social, etc.) on the gradual, but deadly experience of chronic disease across all racial groupings;
3. The social experience of racism and discrimination is indicative of broader cultural dynamics that intersect with and persist in the clinical experiences of women as patients.

In this chapter, we build on the pilot study to integrate and recommend two disciplinary areas in medical research: big data analysis using GIS mapping that has the capacity to coordinate research analyses, clinical training, treatment, and information management between organizations in a region and clinical usage of family diagramming to track and manage more holistic treatment and follow-up for patient-centered care as embedded in family and social contexts including resources, relationships, and other responsibilities that impact on women's health distinctively as indicated by the literature.

Appendix: Providers' Perspective on Women's Experiences in Healthcare

Questionnaire

Our research focuses on the experiences of women as patients in healthcare, and how social determinants of health impact their lives and treatment within clinical and healthcare settings. We would like to ask you several questions about your perspective on women's experiences in healthcare, based on your experience as a professional and practitioner in medical settings.

Your answers to these questions will assist us in situating a somewhat abstract literature review in a "living context" of healthcare delivery, to the extent that there may be overlap or excluded categories.

Please answer as freely and honestly as you can. And, if our scholarship suggests realities that you have not encountered in your experience, or contrasts with your experiences, please do let us know in the answer. It is important that this chapter reflect any gaps between analyses of care and your lived experiences of care toward women as patients, to the extent that we can determine if they exist.

1. What is your current role in which given medical setting(s)?

    (a) How many years of experience have you had in this role?
    (b) In other medical departments or capacities, generally?

2. What has your training been for these roles, cumulatively?
3. Do you believe that women's experiences vary from that of men's, as patients in hospital, clinical, and other medical settings?

    (a) If so, can you provide examples of how?
    (b) If so, do you think the examples of difference occur?
    (c) If so, do you think there are ways that these differences can be addressed? (By your role, in particular?)
    (d) If you do not believe there is much variance, please move on to the next question.

4. In our research, we found that women who live in poverty (or low-income household or neighborhoods) are disproportionately more likely to develop heart disease, diabetes, hypertension, and other major illnesses—across racial groupings. Is it possible for you to observe this occurrence in your experiences with women as patients?

    (a) In what ways are you able to identify the income or educational level of women patients, for example?
    (b) In what ways do you observe the impact of limited economic resources in their experience of healthcare? Or in managing an illness?
    (c) If not, please move on to the next question.

5. Minority women (with few exceptions) were more likely to experience poverty and bias on a regular basis in society. Our research suggests that the experience of racism and discrimination carries over into the clinical experiences of women as patients, too. Have you ever witnessed what you would consider racial bias in treatment?

    (a) If so, in what ways?
    (b) If so, what measures were taken to rectify the situation?
    (c) If not, please move on to the next question.

6. Regarding issues that are specific to women's healthcare (e.g., breast cancer and screening or prevention measures, sexual and reproduction health, maternity care, etc.), do you feel women's healthcare also reveals disparities in the specialized clinical setting?

    (a) If so, what kinds of disparities do you observe in the specialized clinical setting?
    (b) If so, to what do you attribute the disparities that you observe? (For example, are there less resources and staffing? Or, is it the opposite—stark contrasts to the general care units, for example?)

(c) If so, are your observations of disparities also outside of the clinical setting itself? And if so, in what ways? (For example, funding for research? Staffing professionals for care? Health policies? (when it comes to these specialized areas of treatment).

(d) If not, please move on to the next question.

7. Life situations for women in modern society are rather complicated, often as the "Dr. Mom" role can take a toll on women or other role conflicts (as providers and caretakers in multiple family situations) create strain on women's health and ability to manage their own health. In what ways do you observe role strain or role conflict in the way that women experience healthcare as patients?

References

1. Shalowitz, M. U., Schetter, C. D., Hillemeier, M. M., Chinchilli, V. M., Adam, E. K., Hobel, C. J., Ramey, S. L., Vance, M. R., O'Campo, P., Thorp, J. M., Jr., Seeman, T. E., Raju, T., & Eunice Kennedy Shriver National Institute of Child Human Development Community Child Health Network. (2019). Cardiovascular and metabolic risk in women in the first year postpartum: Allostatic load as a function of race, ethnicity, and poverty status. *American Journal of Perinatology, 36*(10), 1079–1089. https://doi.org/10.1055/s-0038-1675618
2. Clarke, A. E. (2014). Biomedicalization. In W. C. Cockerham, R. Dingwall, & S. Quah (Eds.), *The Wiley Blackwell Encyclopedia of health, illness, behavior, and society.* https://doi.org/10.1002/9781118410868.wbehibs083
3. Committee on the Health Professions Education Summit, Institute of Medicine, & Board on Health Care Services. The Core competencies needed for health care professionals. In: Health professions education. National Academies Press. 2003. p. 45–74.
4. Starr, P., & American Council of Learned Societies. (1982). *The social transformation of American medicine (ACLS humanities E-book (series)).* Basic Books.
5. Clarke, A. E., et al. (2010). Biomedicalization technoscience, health, and illness in the U.S. In A. E. Clarke et al. (Eds.), *E-Duke books scholarly collection.* Duke University Press.
6. Agency for Healthcare Research and Quality. (2011) *Health care quality and disparities in women: Selected findings from the 2010 national healthcare quality and disparities reports.*
7. Merzel, C. (2000). Gender differences in health care access indicators in an urban, low-income community. *American Journal of Public Health, 90*(6), 909–916.
8. Kaiser Family Foundation. (2013). *Health reform: Implications for women's access to coverage and care.*
9. Bertakis, K. D., Azari, R., Calhanan, E. J., & Bobbins, J. A. (2000). Gender differences in the utilization of health care services. *The Journal of Family Practice, 49*(2), 147–152.
10. Bronstein, J. M., Felix, H. C., Bursac, Z., Steward, M. K., Foushee, H. R., & Klapow, J. (2012). Providing general and preconception health care to low-income women in family planning settings: Perception of providers and clients. *Maternal Child Health, 16*, 346–354.
11. Salmon, M. M., Joseph, B. M., Saylor, C., & Mann, R. J. (1999). Women's perception of provider, social, and program support in an outpatient drug treatment program. *Journal of Substance Abuse Treatment, 19*(2000), 239–246.
12. Guiahi, M., Sheeder, J., & Teal, S. (2014). Are women aware of religious restrictions on reproductive health at Catholic hospitals? A survey of women's expectations and preferences for family planning care. *Contraception, 90*, 429–434.

13. Trentalange, M., Bielawski, M., Murphy, T. E., Lessard, K., Brandt, C., Bean-Mayberry, B., et al. (2016). Patient perception of enough time spent with provider is a mechanism for improving women veterans' experiences with VA outpatient health care. *Evaluation & The Health Professions, 39*(4), 1–15.
14. Weiss, B. D. (2003). *Health literacy: A manual for clinicians.* American Medical Association Foundation.
15. Ferrari, R. M., Siega-Riz, A. M., Evenson, K. R., Moos, M., & Carrier, K. S. (2012). A qualitative study of women's perceptions of provider advice about diet and physical activity during pregnancy. *Patient Education and Counseling, 91*(2013), 372–377.
16. Heath, C.. American fitness professionals & associates. 2013. Retrieved 06 Jun 2016, from www.afpalfitness.com
17. Haseltine, F. P. (1998). Press 1 for more options. *Journal of Women's Health, 7*(9), 1069–1070.
18. Pitts, C. G. (1999). Women, mental health, and managed care: A disparate system. *Women & Therapy, 22*(3), 27–36.
19. Bridgeman, J. (2007). Exceptional women, healthcare consumers and the inevitability of caring. *Feminist Legal Studies, 15*(2007), 235–245.
20. Close-Up Media (2012). *Trueven Health Analytics— NPR health poll suggests women are more proactive about health screening.*
21. Hucko, D. (2001). Women are key market for healthcare as direct consumers and family influencers. *Marketing to Women, 14*(11).
22. Terplan, M., Longinaker, N., & Appel, L. (2015). Women-centered drug treatment services and need in the United States, 2002–2009. *American Journal of Public Health, 105*(11), e50–e54.
23. Stolp, H., & Fox, J. (2015). Increasing receipt of women's preventive services. *Journal of Women's Health, 24*(11), 875–881.
24. Thabane, L., Ma, J., Chu, R., Cheng, J., Ismaila, A., Rios, L. P., Robson, R., Thabane, M., Giangregorio, L., & Goldsmith, C. H. (2010). A tutorial on pilot studies: The what, why and how. *BMC Medical Research Methodology, 10*, 1. https://doi.org/10.1186/1471-2288-10-1
25. Van Teijlingen, E. R., Rennie, A. M., Hundley, V., & Graham, W. (2001). The importance of conducting and reporting pilot studies: The example of the Scottish births survey. *Journal of Advanced Nursing, 34*, 289–295. https://doi.org/10.1046/j.1365-2648.2001.01757.x
26. Van Teijlingen ER, Hundley V. (2001) The Importance of Pilot Studies. Social Research Update. p. 35:1–4. http://sru.soc.surrey.ac.uk/SRU35.html.
27. Gray, D. (2013). In D. E. Gray (Ed.), *Doing research in the real world* (3rd ed.). SAGE.
28. Blau, F. D., & Kahn, L. M. (2017). The gender wage gap: Extent, trends, and explanations. *Journal of Economic Literature, 55*(3), 789–865.
29. Wasserman, M. (2019). *Hours constraints, occupational choice, and gender: Evidence from medical residents.* Available at SSRN: https://ssrn.com/abstract=3371100 or https://doi.org/10.2139/ssrn.3371100.
30. Cohen, S. A., Sabik, N. J., Cook, S. K., Azzoli, A. B., & Mendez-Luck, C. A. (2019). Differences within differences: gender inequalities in caregiving intensity vary by race and ethnicity in Informa caregivers. *Journal of Cross-Cultural Gerontology, 34*(3), 245–263.
31. Chen, M. (2016). The growing costs and burden of family caregiving of older adults: A review of paid sick leave and family leave policies. *The Gerontologist, 56*(3), 391–396. https://doi.org/10.1093/geront/gnu093
32. Tervalon, M., & Murray-García, J. (1998). Cultural humility versus cultural competence: A critical distinction in defining physician training outcomes in multicultural education. *Journal of Health Care for the Poor and Underserved, 9*(2), 117–125.
33. Women's Health USA 2012, US Department of Health and Human Services. (2013). Available from: https://mchb.hrsa.gov/whusa12/more/introduction.html.
34. Sung, J., Qiu, Q., Marton, J.. New evidence on the relationship between inequality and health. 2019. Available at SSRN: https://ssrn.com/abstract=3174453 or https://doi.org/10.2139/ssrn.3174453

35. Centers for Disease Control and Prevention/Agency for Toxic Substances and Disease Registry/Geospatial Research, Analysis, and Services Program. CDC Social Vulnerability Index 2018 Database US. Accessed 13 Jan 2020.
36. U.S. Cancer Statistics Working Group. U.S. Cancer Statistics Data Visualizations Tool, based on 2019 submission data (1999–2017): U.S. Department of Health and Human Services. Centers for Disease Control and Prevention and National Cancer Institute. www.cdc.gov/cancer/dataviz. Released in June 2020.

Monica D. Griffin, Ph.D. is Director of Engaged Scholarship and the Sharpe Community Scholars Program at William and Mary and an Affiliate Faculty in American Studies. She specializes in community studies, teaching community-based, participatory action research methods, health inequality, and theories of culture, race, and social justice. Monica's research interests include cultural sociology, health inequality (and narrative medicine), and community partnering and action research to study inequality in a variety of organizational settings, including higher education.

Idella G. Glenn, Ph.D. serves as Vice President for Equity, Inclusion, and Community Impact at the University of Southern Maine (USM). Her responsibilities include promoting diversity, equity, and inclusion (DEI) and guiding USM in building a sustainable environment that is inclusive of all faculty, staff, and students. Dr. Glenn has 30 years of experience working in higher education and 25 years of experience in the DEI field.

Chapter 4
The Commoditization of Blacks and the Impact on Health Outcomes

B. DaNine J. Fleming

Silence in the face of injustice not only kills any space for productive conversations, but also allows cancerous ideas to grow. (Jennifer Adaeze Okwerekwu, MD).

Students training to become future healthcare providers and those providing direct patient care must learn not only how to provide quality care, but also how to effectively communicate with patients. The study of cultural issues in healthcare including mental health and an understanding of the effects of race on assessment and treatment is critical to reducing misdiagnosis. To know and consider the effects of race on healthcare can improve physician–patient rapport, and increase levels of patient adherence that can lead to improved patient outcomes. Unconscious bias is an especially relevant factor in suboptimal healthcare services to ethnic minorities, leading to poor communication between a provider and their patient. Communicating with the patient regardless of their cultural background and free of unconscious bias requires introspection, continuous professional development, and training.

There is copious evidence that the quality of physician–patient communication is associated with higher levels of patient satisfaction, better health outcomes, and quality of life [1–7]. The benefit of healthy physician–patient communication is one of the most robust findings in the medical literature. Evidence of its positive impact on patient outcomes dates back about 50 years and extends to racially and culturally diverse patient populations and those with low health literacy [8–12]. However, discernible differences in the quality of physician–patient communication by patient's race and ethnicity have been observed.

A number of studies have reported that differences in race and ethnicity between patients and their providers can represent important cultural barriers to effective communication and partnerships for care. Patient factors such as language barriers,

B. D. J. Fleming (✉)
The Medical University of South Carolina, Diversity, Equity and Inclusion,
Charleston, SC, USA
e-mail: flemid@musc.edu

© The Author(s), under exclusive license to Springer Nature
Switzerland AG 2023
R. Scales, A. T. McCleary-Gaddy (eds.), *Cultural Issues in Healthcare*,
https://doi.org/10.1007/978-3-031-20826-3_4

low health literacy and educational status, and lack of self-efficacy, which may be more prevalent among low-income minorities, may contribute to the risk of poor patient/provider communication in this population [13]. Several factors may impact poor patient/provider communication such as physician factors and healthcare system factors. First, physician factors that may contribute to impaired communication between minority patients and their providers (often from dissimilar race/ethnicity as their patients) include unintentional racial biases in interpreting patient symptoms and decision-making, and poor provider understanding of patients ethnic and cultural disease models and expectations from clinical encounters (Schulman et al. 1999). Next, healthcare system factors may also contribute to poor patient/provider communication, for example, by placing overly restrictive time constraints on the healthcare encounter or by failing to have culturally and literacy-appropriate educational materials available for use by healthcare professionals [13].

Communication is essential for the patient to communicate the severity of his or her illness, as well as for the healthcare provider to instruct patients on pharmacologic and nonpharmacologic care. Communication problems stem from issues with patients, healthcare providers, and healthcare systems (CHEST 2007). A comprehensive search using the PRISMA guidelines was conducted across seven online databases between 1995 and 2016 and results found that Results indicated that black patients consistently experienced poorer communication quality, information-giving, patient participation, and participatory decision-making than white patients [14]. "Extensive research has shown that no matter how knowledgeable a clinician might be, if he or she is not able to open good communication with a patient, he or she may be of no help" [15]. Patients' perceptions of the quality of the healthcare they received are highly dependent on the quality of their interactions with their healthcare clinician and team.

According to Dr. Robert Pearl [16], "The US lags behind other industrialized nations in many important health measures—partly because citizens of certain races, ethnicities, and incomes experience poorer versions of US healthcare than others. The disparities are glaring." One reason the United States ranks so poorly globally is that health outcomes for certain racial, ethnic, and socioeconomic groups fare so poorly domestically. African Americans, Latinos, and the economically disadvantaged experience poorer healthcare access and lower quality of care than white Americans, and in most measures, that gap is growing [16]. According to a 2014 report from the Robert Wood Johnson Foundation (RWJ), "your healthcare depends on who you are. Race and ethnicity continue to influence a patient's chances of receiving many specific healthcare interventions and treatments." The RWJ Foundation is the nation's largest philanthropy dedicated to health.

Definitions

In an effort to ensure a consistent frame of reference for the terms utilized throughout this chapter, pervasive terms are defined below.

Commoditization can be defined as the process by which goods that have economic value and are distinguishable in terms of attributes (uniqueness or brand) end up becoming simple commodities in the eyes of the market or consumers [17]. The action or process of treating something as a mere commodity.

Commoditization is a generalized Darwinian selection pressure in economic evolution driven by profit-and-efficiency-seeking in the investment of key resources. By winnowing non-commodity opportunities to satisfy human needs, commoditization distorts development in ways that intensify negative social outcomes experienced by oppressed groups and undermines the possibility for sustainable development [18].

Ecological economics is a growing transdisciplinary field that aims to improve and expand economic theory to integrate the earth's natural systems, human values, and human health and well-being.

Ecosystems—a biological community of interacting organisms and their physical environment (in general use) a complex network or interconnected system.

Existential violence—existing violence.

Oppression—systematic mistreatment which includes not only material inequalities of access and privilege but also deprivation of recognition, appreciation, understanding, and other forms of "inclusion necessary for groups and communities to flourish" (p. 732) [19].

Quality—According to The Institute of Medicine, quality is defined as "the degree to which health services for individuals and populations increase the likelihood of desired health outcomes and are consistent with current professional knowledge" [20].

Unconscious Bias—also known as, implicit bias, is the bias in judgment and/or behavior that results from subtle cognitive processes that often operate at a level below conscious awareness and without intentional control [21].

White Coat Anxiety/White Coat Syndrome/White Coat Hypertension—is a phenomenon in which patients exhibit a blood pressure level above the normal range, in a clinical setting, though they do not exhibit it in other settings. It is believed that the phenomenon is due to anxiety that those afflicted experience during a clinic visit [22].

White Fragility—a state in which even a minimum amount of racial stress becomes intolerable, triggering a range of defensive moves [23].

> If we swim against the "current" of racial privilege, it's often easier to recognize, while harder to recognize if we swim with it. (Robin DiAngelo)

Accountability

Manno [18] states "when oppression is conceptualized as a result of maldevelopment, then the remedies involve social and economic change. The remedy is not only the inclusion of the excluded into the benefits derived from the major productive activities of the economy, but also the deliberate expansion of investment toward those socially essential but economically "inefficient" goods and services that are embodied in relationships. He further asserts that certain groups of people, as a result of their history, personal experience, and/or cultural and political resistance to commoditization, and/or because of their close ties to sectors of the economy with low commodity potential, receive disproportionately smaller shares of resources. As this disproportionate allocation accumulates over time, the result is a palpable experience of being underprivileged. Cultural identity is integral to all aspects of life and is a constitutive facet of self-identity. The degree to which healthcare providers are culturally aware can shape patients' ability to receive and apply information regarding their own healthcare, which consequently affects overall health [24–26]. However, if and when an educational program does directly address racism and the privileging of whites, the common white response includes anger, withdrawal, emotional incapacitation, guilt, argumentation, and cognitive dissonance (all of which reinforce the pressure on facilitators to avoid directly addressing racism) [23]. So-called progressive whites may not respond with anger, but may still insulate themselves via claims that they are beyond the need for engaging with the content because they "already had a class on this" or "already know this." These reactions are often seen in anti-racist education endeavors as forms of resistance to the challenge of internalized dominance ([27–29], O'Donnell 1998). These responses are evident in 2020 during the national COVID-19 pandemic and with the racial unrest with the call for Federal agencies to cease and desist from using taxpayer dollars to fund diversity and inclusion training that is considered by the current administration to be "divisive, un-American propaganda that includes critical race theory, white privilege or any other training or propaganda."

White Fragility is a state in which even a minimum amount of racial stress becomes intolerable, triggering a range of defensive moves. Fine [30] identifies this insulation when she observes "… how Whiteness accrues privilege and status; gets itself surrounded by protective pillows of resources and/or benefits of the doubt; how Whiteness repels gossip and voyeurism and instead demands dignity" (p. 57). Whites are rarely without these "protective pillows," and when they are, it is usually temporary and by choice. This insulated environment of racial privilege builds white expectations for racial comfort while at the same time lowering the ability to tolerate racial stress. The American feminist and anti-racism activist Peggy McIntosh [31] states, "Whites are taught to see their perspectives as objective and representative of reality." Whiteness is not recognized or named by white people, and a universal reference point is assumed. White people are just people. Within this construction, whites can represent humanity; meanwhile, non-white people, who are never just people but always most particularly black people, Asian people, etc., can only represent their own racialized experiences [32]. This is particularly problematic in healthcare because this disassociation between explicit and implicit attitudes shapes the behaviors and perceptions of interracial interactions leading not only to the Black-White perception gap but fueling the miscommunications and misunderstandings that continue to perpetuate racial tensions [33], and can also perpetuate racial tensions aid in healthcare disparities alike. Populations that experience health disparities include racial and ethnic minority groups, socioeconomically disadvantaged groups, and rural populations (National Center for Minority Health and Health Disparities 2003).

> "When doctors communicate with patients, there's a series of unspoken choices they make-what to say and what not to say, who to include in important discussions, what counsel to provide, and what kind of follow-up care is needed. Many of these communication decisions may be influenced by assumptions and stereotypes about who a patient is, what "their story" is, and what their goals are. If the assumptions are wrong, it can limit a patient's choices and compromise a patient's health" (Barnes, 2013).

A Culture of Distrust: The Impact on Health Outcomes

According to Young [34], "those groups of people who have been hurt the most by oppression and have gained the least from the benefits of commoditization—indigenous people and other people of color, women, people with disabilities, and everyone who has only their labor to sell (working-class people)—are the targets of racism, sexism, classism, and disability oppression." Given the knowledge of past experiences in healthcare, there are legitimate reasons for distrust. According to [35], distrust is ubiquitous in all facets of the research enterprise and extended from members of the research and medical communities (Skinner et al. 2015; Drake et al. 2017; Kraft et al. 2018), to medical or research institutions (Drake et al. 2017; Kraft et al. 2018), and the conduct of research and science in general (Skinner et al. 2015). The Tuskegee Study of Untreated Syphilis which is discussed later in this chapter at length, frequently functioned as a historical referent for the distrust of biomedical research, particularly among African Americans.

Because the problem is multifaceted, the solutions must be as well [16]. It remains the perception of the medical community that Tuskegee accounts for the distrust of the healthcare system and clinical trials in particular [36]. However, the distrust of the medical community extends far beyond the Tuskegee experiment and is based not only on historical injustices that go back generations, but also on the continued structural racism that is part of the current reality [36, 37]. Research on Black attitudes and beliefs continues to document that Blacks from all educational levels hold a distrust of a medical system that is dominated by the White society [38–44]. Routinely, participants in these studies discussed feelings of not being understood (cultural values, beliefs, and life situations), feelings of being treated without respect and used as "guinea pigs" for White students; and their feelings that the White establishment was responsible for purposely infecting the Black communities with AIDS and illegal drugs [45, 46].

Cose [47] chronicles the rage of successful Blacks who find themselves constantly assaulted by a hostile environment while having to maintain a silent struggle or be labeled as the problem. In Carroll's [48] research, a 17-years old describes what it was like to be Black, "Nobody has done anything wrong here, but it's like having to work at a job I didn't apply for. I alone have to come up with the added strength to deal with racism" (p. 53). Black people are tired of being seen as Black first and a person second. The persistence of this feeling is reflected in the 1903 writings of W.E.B. DuBois, whose *The Souls of Black Folks*, would become the classical foundation of the sociological study of Blacks in America. In this narrative, he attempts to answer the question, "how does it feel to be the problem?"

> It is a peculiar sensation, this double-consciousness, this sense of always looking at one's self through the eyes of others, of measuring one's soul by the tape of a world that looks on in amused contempt and pity. One ever feels his twoness-an American, a Negro; two souls, two thoughts, two unreconciled strivings; two warring ideals in one dark body, whose dogged strength alone keeps it from being torn asunder [49]: 215.

In the Black community, they refer to the exhaustion from this "added strength" as suffering from "White People Fatigue Syndrome" [50]: 177. In this country, the lived social reality of African American individuals is experienced through the color of their skin. Their identity is bound by the racial inequities of our society. It has been suggested that the emotions of anger and frustration resulting from this institutionalized racial discrimination are an emotional causative pathway to the pathophysiology that we now know contributes to the health disparities experienced by African Americans [33].

Beliefs that blacks and whites are fundamentally and biologically different have been prevalent in various forms for centuries. As described by the earlier examples, these beliefs were championed by scientists, physicians, and slave owners alike to justify slavery and the inhumane treatment of black men and women in medical research [51–53], Hoffman et al. (2015). Recent research reveals that a substantial number of white laypeople and medical students and residents continue to hold false beliefs about biological differences between blacks and whites and that these beliefs predict racial bias in pain perception and influence the accuracy of treatment recommendations generally, but notably in pain treatment recommendations [54]. Extant research has shown that, relative to white patients, black patients are less likely to be given pain medications and, if given pain medications, they receive lower quantities [55, 56], Smedley et al. (2013).

Today, many laypeople, scientists, and scholars continue to believe that the black body is biologically and fundamentally different from the white body and that race is a fixed marker of group membership, rooted in biology [54]. In fact, many people insist that black people are better athletes—stronger, faster, and more agile— as a result of natural selection and deliberate breeding practices during slavery [57–59]. Research suggests that people even believe that black people are more likely than white people to be capable of fantastical mental and physical feats, such as withstanding extreme heat from burning coals [60]. These biological conceptions of race are only weakly if at all correlated with racial attitudes [61, 62]. They are nonetheless consequential. Research has shown that biological conceptions and related beliefs are associated with greater acceptance of racial disparities [62] and even racial bias in pain perception [63]. The distrust of White society is so great that conspiracy theories are common, particularly in areas that intersect with the White healthcare establishment [45, 46, 64, 65].

According to Increasing Diversity in the U.S.: The Importance of Cultural Competence in Healthcare in Medcom (2016), a lack of diversity in the healthcare workforce and its leadership is among the leading barriers to cultural competence, contributing to racial and ethnic disparities of care. Poorly designed care systems that fail to meet the needs of all patient populations, and poor communication between providers and patients of different racial, cultural, and ethnic backgrounds are additional barriers. This last year marks the 35th anniversary of the landmark 1985 Report of the Secretary's Task Force on Black and Minority Health, more commonly known as the Heckler Report. This report, the first comprehensive documentation of racial disparities in health by medical experts, put a national spotlight on the pervasive racial inequities in health and issued a resounding call to eliminate health disparities. Although this call was met with a surge in research efforts and substantial changes in medical programs, policy, and legislation, the ultimate goal of eliminating racial disparities remains elusive.

Healthcare Disparities

Understanding the Black-White dynamic is only a first step in shifting the underlying assumptions of health and health disparities research. The challenge now is to move beyond documenting that racial health disparities exist to explanations that challenge the status quo. This calls for a revision in our paradigms of knowledge generation regarding race, health, truth, and power [33]. Since health disparities continue to persist, more effective strategies for their reduction and elimination must be considered, developed, and implemented. One such strategy is the incorporation of healthcare workforce development and training programs to promote diversity. Given the higher prevalence of disparate care in racial and ethnic minority groups, such as Non-Hispanic Blacks (NHB), Hispanics, and American Indians/ Alaskan Natives (AIAN), it is strategic to promote diversity in the workforce by promoting diversity during recruitment and training [66].

To better understand Black health disparities, it is also necessary to shift the paradigms of disease risk to an integrated framework that considers both the cumulative effects of the life course and the cumulative effects of multiple layers of physiological stress. An integrated, cumulative perspective provides a significantly different picture of risk, resilience, and disease [33].

According to an article in Families USA, "African American health disparities compared to Non-Hispanic Whites," the only way to reduce racial and ethnic health disparities is to work together to improve our healthcare system to make it high quality, comprehensive, affordable, and accessible for everyone (2014). Despite the fact that the great majority of healthcare providers abhor prejudice and make every effort to deliver healthcare that is fair and equal to all patients, the Institute of Medicine report [67] concluded that the preponderance of evidence suggests that inadvertent bias, stereotyping, prejudice, and clinical uncertainty are likely important contributing factors to healthcare disparities. [13].

Research by Dovidio et al. [68] focused on the subtle, contemporary form of racial prejudice and bias that characterizes and contributes to the perception gap between Blacks and Whites. What these researchers term "aversion racism" relies on both explicit (conscious) and implicit (unconscious) attitudes that influence behavior. Brooks [69] writes, "if we refuse to deeply examine and challenge how racism and implicit bias affect our clinical practice, we will continue to contribute to health inequities in a way that will remain unaddressed in our curriculum and unchallenged by future generations of physicians." According to the results of a study utilizing cultural sensitivity training by Majumdar et al. [70], there are tremendous benefits of promoting cultural awareness among healthcare providers in terms of reducing cultural disparities in the healthcare system. The success of such programs demonstrates that if we want to change the system we must be willing to acknowledge that there is a problem within the system. Brooks [69] writes, "if we refuse to deeply examine and challenge how racism and implicit bias affect our clinical practice, we will continue to contribute to health inequities in a way that will remain unaddressed in our curriculum and unchallenged by future generations of physicians."

Racial and ethnic health disparities are undermining our communities and our health system. African Americans are more likely to suffer from certain health conditions, and they are more likely to get sicker, have serious complications, and even die from them. According to statistics gathered by Families USA (April 2014), some of the more common health disparities that affect African Americans in the United States compared to non-Hispanic whites in adults include, but are not limited to depression (20% less likely to receive treatment for depression), stroke (40% more likely to die from stroke), heart disease (30% more likely to die of heart disease), obesity (40% more likely to be obese), maternal mortality (x2.5 as likely to die during pregnancy), prostate cancer (x2 as likely to die from prostate cancer), cervical cancer (x2 as likely to die from cervical cancer), breast cancer (40% more likely to die from breast cancer), asthma (x2.1 as likely to die from asthma), HIV (x9 as likely to be diagnosed with HIV, x8 as likely to die from HIV), and diabetes (60% more likely to be diabetic, x2 as likely to undergo leg, foot, or toe amputation). Improved health professions education is one of the critical and potentially most effective interventions to eliminate healthcare disparities [71]. We must work to optimize the best outcomes for all patients and populations.

History of the Commoditization of Blacks

Rather than a historical stage, industrial capitalism should be understood as a function of specialization within a larger field of accumulation strategies (p. 172). The phenomenon of commoditization operates whenever dominant elites extract economic surplus, not for reinvestment in economic development beneficial to the producers (peasants or workers), but for consumption or investment elsewhere. Being "elsewhere," the elites are buffered from the environmental and social consequences. Thus, the distortion of development will occur under all forms of economic domination and oppression as both dominant and dominated and/or rational strategies for the allocation of the resources to best thrive or at least survive in the situations in which they find themselves. These strategies are internalized and provide behavior-determining cues, even when they are damaging to the full flourishing of one's humanness. This is what is meant by internalized oppression. [72]

According to Manno [18], commoditization leads to the underdevelopment of the economy of relationships and overdevelopment of the economy of things. Accordingly, what we call highly developed societies could, he suggests, be described as societies whose development patterns have been highly distorted by the logic and values of markets through the process of commoditization. This distortion of development has profound consequences for human well-being and should and can be an important subject for ecological economics. Leopold [73] explained that when we unwittingly undermine the integrity of ecosystems we undermine the health of everything that is a part of the ecosystem, including ourselves. Empathy, morality, and love for others is the glue that holds human societies together [74].

Although medical experimentation with human subjects has historically involved vulnerable groups, including children and the poor and the institutionalized, black Americans have disproportionately borne the burden of the most invasive, inhumane, and perilous medical investigations, from the era of slavery to the present day [75]. Some examples of medical experimentation include the Tuskegee Syphilis Study and the story of Henrietta Lacks.

In the case of the Tuskegee Syphilis Study, the military covertly tested mustard gas and other chemicals on black soldiers during World War II, and the US Public Health Service, in collaboration with the Tuskegee Institute, studied the progression of untreated syphilis in black men from 1932 to 1972. The Tuskegee Syphilis Study is still recognized today as one of the most notorious cases of prolonged and knowing violation of human subjects, according to a report "Why African Americans May Not Be Participating in Clinical Trials (1996)." The study involved mostly poor, illiterate Blacks who were infected with syphilis. "The study was designed to document the natural history of syphilis," the report states. More specifically, researchers wanted to observe how the disease progressed differently in blacks in its late stages and to examine its devastating effects with postmortem dissection. One of the main ethical issues, though there were many with this study, was the fact that participants were neither given penicillin once it emerged as a standard treatment for syphilis in the 1930s nor were they made aware that there were effective treatment options for the disease [43]. This tragic 40-year-long public health project resulted in almost 400 impoverished and unsuspecting African American men in Macon County, Alabama being left untreated for syphilis [75]. Washington [75] states, "there is a pervasive history of exploitation of black subjects in U.S. medical research. Tuskegee was the longest and most infamous—but hardly the worst—experimental abuse of African Americans. It has been eclipsed in both numbers and egregiousness by other abusive medical studies."

Another infamous case is that of Henrietta Lacks, whom scientists refer to even today as "HeLa." Lacks was a poor black tobacco farmer whose cells—taken without her knowledge or permission in 1951—became the source of the first line of immortal human cells and one of the most important tools in medicine as they proved vital for developing polio vaccine, cloning, gene mapping, in vitro fertilization, and more. When doctors noticed that Lacks' cells were able to stay alive for longer periods of time than previous cells, they removed two samples of her cervix during surgery—one part that was healthy and one part that was cancerous [76]—in order to conduct research on the cell composition. Since their collection, researchers have grown roughly 20 tons of her cells. In addition to harvesting Lacks' cells without her knowledge or permission, researchers also published the family's medical records without their consent. Henrietta's cells have been bought and sold by the billions, yet she remains virtually unknown, and her family continues to live in poverty today. The situation for indigenous peoples (any group whose ways of life have coevolved over extensive periods of time in a particular ecosystem) is directly related to the effects of commoditization which undervalue an important component of their very being, their connection with the ecosystem [18].

There are also documented examples of reproductive commoditization of Blacks. According to Jayawardene [77], at the heart of colonial slavery was White masters' ability to exert control over Black women's reproductive labor. In 1662, when Virginia enacted a law differentiating enslavement from indentured servitude, the status of mulatto offspring was determined based on the condition of the mother, marking a dramatic departure from English common law wherein the condition of the father determined the legal status of children [78]. This law transformed Black women's reproductive capacity into the means through which slave property was sustained and produced [79]. Later, following the ban on slave importation in 1808, the enslaved labor force was replenished through Black women's childbearing capacities, which effectively became "subject to social regulation rather than their own will" ([80], pp. 22–23). This was the use of legal means to legitimize and standardize the commoditization of Black women's reproductive labor.

Under slavery, not only did the Black family offer a sound and dependable source of new laborers Black women also reproduced cheap labor while they worked in the fields and nurtured and fed their own families [81]. To secure Black women's reproductive labor, slave owners adopted varying degrees of intimidating approaches. According to Flavin [82], some offered incentives like a lighter workload or extra rations to pregnant slaves, some were spared harsh disciplinary action during pregnancy, and some women were allowed easier working conditions; (although many accounts indicate they were expected to continue performing strenuous fieldwork). In more rare instances, masters would grant permanent freedom from fieldwork to women who had already birthed a required number of children" [82]. All of the slave masters' strategies are consistent with what Ani [83] termed "commoditized oppression" and the persistence of violence in the contemporary birthing contexts of Black women.

In the nineteenth century, prominent physicians sought to establish the "physical peculiarities" of blacks that could "serve to distinguish from the white man" [53]. Such "peculiarities" included thicker skin, less sensitive nervous systems. And diseases inherent in dark skin [51, 84]. Dr. Samuel Cartwright, for instance, wrote that blacks bore a "Negro disease (making them) insensible to pain when subjected to punishment" [51]. Other physicians believed that blacks could tolerate surgical operations with little, if any, pain at all [52, 75]. Well into the twentieth century, researchers continued to experiment on black people based in part on the assumption that the black body was more resistant to pain and injury. In 1855, the escaped slave John "Fed" Brown recalled that the doctor to whom he was indentured produced painful blisters on his body in order to observe "how deep my black skin went" (Brown, 1854, pp. 48). Mr. Brown's experience was one of an innumerable and largely unreported "studies" that held no therapeutic value. Rather, fascination with the outward appearance of African Americans, whose differences from whites were thought to be more than skin deep, was a significant impulse driving such medical trials throughout slavery.

Shielding whites from excruciating experimental procedures also proved a powerful motivation for which enslaved Black people were subjected to countless cruel and inhuman medical studies and experiments. Perhaps one of the most famous examples came from J. Marion Sims who still hail as the "Father of Modern Gynecology" [85]. Born in Lancaster County, South Carolina, Sims conducted multiple experiments on enslaved women in order to treat vesicovaginal fistula, a condition that caused a great deal of pain. Sims performed surgeries on the women without using any anesthesia because he believed the operations were not "painful enough to justify the trouble," he said during a lecture in 1857. Given Sim's practices among slaves in the mid-nineteenth century ([86, 87], Harris 1950), he was among the first doctors of the modern era to emphasize women's health, and both his patients' then—and countless thousands of women since—benefited from his success.

Few can argue with the historical significance of slavery and Jim Crow laws on the oppression and segregation of Black people of African American ancestry [33]. Jim Crow laws maintained racial segregation in the South beginning in the late 1800s. After slavery ended, many whites feared the freedom of blacks. They loathed the idea that it would be possible for African Americans to achieve the same social status as whites if given the same access to employment, healthcare, housing, and education. Already uncomfortable with the gains some blacks made during Reconstruction, whites took issue with such a prospect. As a result, states began to pass laws that placed a number of restrictions on blacks. Collectively, these laws limited black advancement and ultimately gave blacks the status of second-class citizens. Racial apartheid in the United States soon earned the nickname, Jim Crow [88]. The ethnocentrism of Whiteness as a norm comes with a certain set of assumptions that often remain unexamined. These are the everyday assumptions of neutrality, superiority, and dominance [89]. Ethnocentrism is the belief that one's own way of life or culture is superior to others. The implicit notion here is that what is normal for us is preferable in general and what is unfamiliar is less good [90].

It has been 35 years since the landmark 1985 *Report of the Secretary's Task Force on Black and Minority Health*—commonly known as the *Heckler*

Report—the first comprehensive documentation of racial disparities in health by medical experts. This report put a national spotlight on the pervasive racial inequities in health and issues a resounding call to eliminate health disparities. This study demonstrates that beliefs about biological differences between blacks and whites— beliefs dating back to slavery—are associated with the perception that black people feel less pain than white people and with inadequate treatment recommendations for black patients' pain.

The relevance is reflected in the racial bias in pain assessment study conducted by Hoffman et al. (2015) and shows how Black Americans are systematically under-treated for pain relative to white Americans even in the twenty-first century. The study examined whether this racial bias is related to false beliefs about biological differences between blacks and whites (e.g., "black people's skin is thicker than white people's skin). This research provides evidence that white laypeople and medical students and residents believe that the black body is biologically differ-ent—and in many cases, stronger—than the white body. Moreover, they provide evidence that these beliefs are associated with racial bias in perceptions of others' pain, which in turn predict accuracy in pain treatment recommendations. The cur-rent work addresses an important social factor that may contribute to racial bias in health and healthcare.

Sabin [91] states:

> Racial and ethnic disparities in pain treatment are not intentional. Instead, inequities are the product of complex influences, including implicit biases that providers don't even know they have. As a nation, we must continue to reckon with the lingering history of racism in medicine. We in academic medicine have a duty to bring to light racist misinformation, stereotypes, and unconscious attitudes that contribute to disparities in patient care today. Dramatically reducing, and perhaps even eliminating, racial and ethnic disparities in pain treatment is an attainable goal — and a moral imperative.

Communication

> The problem with communication is the illusion that it has occurred.—George Bernard Shaw

The effort to foster effective communication among healthcare providers and with patients and families is a significant challenge in our complex healthcare systems [92]. Most complaints by patients and the public about doctors deal with problems of communication not with clinical competency [93]. The most common complaint is that doctors do not listen to them. In addition, patients want more and better infor-mation about their problem and the outcome, more openness about the side effects of treatment, relief of pain and emotional distress, and advice on what they can do for themselves [94]. Several studies have shown that doctors and patients have dif-ferent views on what makes good and effective communication [95]. These differ-ences influence the quality of interactions between doctors and patients, as well as compliance, patient education, and health outcomes [94]. A comprehensive search using the PRISMA guidelines was conducted across seven online databases between 1995 and 2016 and results found that Results indicated that black patients consistently experienced poorer communication quality, information-giving, patient participation, and participatory decision-making than white patients [14]. Patients today are health consumers and want to be active participants in medical decision-making. Good doctor–patient communication offers patients tangible benefits. Many studies have found significant positive associations between doctors' communication skills and patients' satisfaction [2]. Several studies and reviews also show a correlation between effective communication and improved health outcomes [3]. High-quality interpersonal relationships, communication, and "whole person" knowledge of patients have been correlated with improvements in clinical and functional adherence, patient trust, reduced malpractice suits, and satisfaction of both physicians and patients with their encounters [3, 96–98].

Dr. Harlan Krumholz [99], a cardiologist and Harold H. Hines, Jr. professor of medicine and epidemiology and public health at the Yale School of Medicine at Yale University states:

> "I have always thought that the conversations with patients have the potential to be therapeutic or harmful. We can promote the kind of communication that enables patients to be better able to make difficult choices, to be more confident in pursuing the strategies they choose and to be more likely to achieve the results that they desire. And we need to avoid the kind of communication that alienates patients from the health-care system, inhibits them from honestly disclosing how they feel and what they need, interferes with their ability to make the choices that best fit them and reduces the likelihood that they will get the outcomes they desire."

According to Increasing Diversity in the U.S.: The Importance of Cultural Competence in Healthcare in Medcom (2016), respect is at the heart of cultural competence-patients who feel their healthcare providers respect their beliefs, customs, values, language, and traditions are more likely to communicate freely and honestly, which can, in turn, reduce disparities in healthcare and improve patient outcomes. Sadly, although the loss of respect for the power of connecting with patients is not the fault of doctors, it seems to be a byproduct of the medical environment that we have created and the behaviors that we reward [99]. Although medical educators and clinicians strive to create positive learning environments, the "hidden curriculum," that which is learned by watching what teachers and clinicians do rather than by merely listening to what they say, continues to undermine compassion, collaboration, and communication [100, 101]. Unfortunately, the medical community has not systematically addressed the need to foster, teach, and evaluate communication and collaboration with patients among professionals across the continuum of health profession education [102].

The manner in which information is communicated to patients can also influence their perceptions of the healthcare system and can affect their adherence to prescribed healthcare regimens [70]. According to Fred Hassan (2013), Chairman of Bausch & Lomb, "the single biggest thing is to have empathy and to actively listen and communicate. Doctors are not taught the importance of this skill very well in school." Studies show that up to 80% of the medical information patients receive is forgotten immediately and nearly half of the information retained is incorrect. To ensure patients understand and remember critical information about their treatment and healthcare plans, their doctor can ask her or him to describe the plan in their own words, a strategy utilized known as the teach-back method. The goal of good communication should be getting the best outcomes for patients. Seen in that light, the key for doctors improving their communication with patients is the quality of their communication with fellow clinicians, states Leah Binder (2013), president and CEO of LeapFrog Group. She goes on to state, "Good medicine is a team sport. Good team communication is life or death for patients."

Case for Additional Education and Training

Manno [18] asserts, "an oppressed group is made up of individuals who may or may not share other things in common but they have in common a set of identifiable shared experiences of deprivation of development capabilities. Because much of what oppressed people experience is often a result of a direct and personal abuse of economic, political, or personal power, it is those aspects of oppression that have received the most attention." For many white people, a single required multicultural education course taken in college, or required "cultural competency training" in their workplace, is the only time they may encounter a direct and sustained challenge to their racial understandings. But even in this arena, not all multicultural courses or training programs talk directly about racism, much less address white privilege. It is far more than the norm for these courses and programs to use racially coded language such as "urban," "inner city," and "disadvantaged" but to rarely use "white" or "over advantaged" or "privileged."

Frankenberg [103] defines Whiteness as multidimensional:

> Whiteness is a location of structural advantage, of race privilege. Second, it is a 'standpoint,' a place from which White people look at ourselves, at others, and at society. Third, 'Whiteness' refers to a set of cultural practices that are usually unmarked and unnamed. (p.1)

Further, white people are taught not to feel any loss over the absence of people of color in their lives and in fact, this absence is what defines their schools and neighborhoods as "good" whites come to understand that a "good school" or "good neighborhood" is coded language for "white" [104]. Meryn [94] states there is evidence that supports changing doctors' behavior and communication skills can be achieved quite easily with proper teaching [2, 105, 106].

Meryn goes on to say that the practice of medicine is more than a job. It requires doctors to have a moral and social responsibility as well as a medical responsibility and must preserve their patients' trust. Finally, he states that communication is an interactive process that requires patients to have skills and support to take part in decision-making and raise questions about quality. Govere & Govere [107] conducted a systematic review to evaluate the literature on how effective cultural competence training was in improving cultural competence levels of healthcare providers and to determine whether the trained healthcare providers increased patient satisfaction among clients from minority groups. They found that the seven studies exhibited a high degree of variability. They differed on experimental designs, intervention and patient participants, intervention treatments (e.g., cultural competence training content, duration, and methods), cultural competence and patient satisfaction assessment tools, and intervention outcomes (whether cultural competence training increased cultural competence levels and consequently patient satisfaction). Although there were shortcomings, the studies agreed that cultural competence training was associated with improved cultural competence of healthcare providers and increased patient satisfaction. Therefore, there is a need for healthcare specialties to develop and introduce provider-targeted cultural competence training protocols and evaluate their impact on cultural competence levels of healthcare providers and patient satisfaction using specialized valid and reliable standardized assessment tools.

Path Forward

"Your health care depends on who you are," according to a 2014 report from the Robert Wood Johnson Foundation, the nation's largest philanthropy dedicated to health. "Race and ethnicity continue to influence a patient's chances of receiving many specific healthcare interventions and treatments." This can no longer be the case. Fraser [108] argues that institutionalized norms associated with dominant values have the effect of excluding those with an alternative of conflicting norms from participation. Both of these views suggest that in considering the effects of commoditization on those people whose cultural values give priority to relationships (human and ecological) we should look at the impacts of institutionalized patterns of allocation on people's capabilities for participation in development. Lown and Manning [92] assert few opportunities exist to enhance relationships and communication among all members of multidisciplinary healthcare teams, to teach the advanced communication skills needed in our complex healthcare environments, and to create supportive environments in which all can learn from each other. This must change to optimize care.

According to Dr. Atul Grover (2013), chief public policy officer of the Association of American Medical Colleges, medical schools and teaching hospitals are working with schools of nursing and pharmacy to educate and train health professionals in interprofessional teams. It is their belief that this team approach will reshape medical practice in the future and help all caregivers do a better job of listening to patients.

As the United States continues to recover from a global pandemic, racial unrest due to continued police brutality and White supremacy, the Trump administration issued a recent memorandum directing that training of employees in federal agencies on diversity, equity, and inclusion cease. There is no way to ignore this elephant in the room. At a minimum, these educational opportunities are designed to explore the differences that range from social identities that are impacted by these federal agencies' work to intuitional racism that is a part of the history of the United States. It is undeniable that racism and systemic oppression is deeply embedded in US history, and this nation was built on colonization, slavery, and violence perpetrated against the most marginalized individuals namely African Americans and Indigenous people. To continue to deny this is to deny history.

In a memorandum, written by Russel Vought, Director of the Office of Management and Budget (September 4, 2020), Vought stated that "The President has directed me to ensure that Federal agencies cease and desist from using taxpayer dollars to fund these divisive, un-American propaganda training sessions. Accordingly, to that end, the Office of Management and Budget will shortly issue more detailed guidance on implementing the President's directive. In the meantime, all agencies are directed to begin to identify all contracts or other agency spending related to any training on "critical race theory," "white privilege," or any other training or propaganda effort that teaches or suggests either (1) that the United States is an inherently racist or evil country or (2) that any race or ethnicity is inherently racist or evil. In addition, all agencies should begin to identify all available avenues within the law to cancel any such contracts and/or to divert Federal dollars away from these un-American propaganda training sessions."

Let us not be confused that this directive was issued at a time when our country is engaged in a national shift that has been reignited by groups such as Black Lives Matter, Colin Kaepernick, and other organizations demanding justice for all Americans with a particular focus on Black Americans who are being disproportionately harmed. And with such travesties as the deaths of Botham Jean, George Floyd, Ahmaud Arbury, Breonna Taylor, and countless others, we know the time is now and there is no time for retreat we must move forward with all deliberate speed. We are a precious commodity and Black lives DO matter.

From the words of the National Association of Diversity Officers in Higher Education (NADOHE):

> As a country, we are confronted with racism's violence and dangerous consequences, and, in good conscience, we cannot tolerate this violence and inequity. As a society, we are compelled to end the discrimination and systems of oppression that allows unequal opportunities, senseless violence, and even death. There has also been an awakening in every state of this union and higher education, particularly as it welcomes students back in the fall that Anti-Blackness has permeated every sector of our society. The COVID-19 pandemic has devastated Black, Brown, and Indigenous communities, from infection and death rates to access to quality health care, high unemployment rates, the risks associated with being essential workers, and housing and economic insecurity. At this time of racial reckoning with our past, the President deepens the divide and eliminates any possibility that individuals within the federal government can learn the consequences of racism and its deadly effects. Worse yet, it is a signal to our citizens and the world that racism does not exist and never existed. Eliminating these critical conversations on race is an erasure of history at a time when we need this understanding more than ever to transform our society into a just

one. Doing away with DEI education and development designed to foster dialogue on race and the effects of structural racism is unfathomable. More than ever, our country needs dialogue and facilitated DEI workshops. Recalling this commitment does not make one more American or patriotic. On the contrary, we cannot think of anything more American than to fight for justice, freedom, and equality. It is also patriotic to own up to our failings to create a better country, right past wrongs, and build our capacity as Americans to work together. As a country, we strive to be a shining example to the world of what a shared democracy governed by the people for the people truly means. NADOHE urges higher education to continue and strengthen its existing commitment to racial equity and DEI workshops, seminars, courses, and lectures that explore racism in all its harsh reality. We cannot fix the scourge of racism if we negate its existence. We cannot end violence against the Black community and other minoritized groups if we do not foster dialogue and understanding. We cannot welcome our students without addressing structural racism. It is our responsibility to prepare our students to work and live in a diverse society. We cannot accomplish this goal if we cannot discuss race and work toward ending structural racism. As the pre-eminent voice for chief diversity officers in higher education and with more than 1,100 members representing 750 colleges and universities, NADOHE's mission is to lead higher education towards inclusive excellence through institutional transformation.

In conclusion, if the change is to be effectual and sustainable we first must acknowledge that there is a systemic issue that needs to be addressed. We must then be willing to make the time to provide additional comprehensive education and training. Finally, we must be willing to hold all individuals accountable regardless of position or status. The most important thing we can do is to remind our clinicians—and teach our students—that the real patient is important, and that the human connection is essential to the art of healing, and every patient we see, is observing our every move for signals that we actually care about what happens to them [109]. We still have much to learn about the cultural barriers that prevent some patients from obtaining the best possible healthcare. But that alone will not be enough to make a difference. We must agree that unequal care is unacceptable. Only then can we make all of the improvements our nation needs [16].

References

1. Nouri, S., & Rudd, R. (2015). Health literacy in the "oral exchange": An important element of patient-provider communication. *Patient Education and Counseling, 98*, 565–571. https://doi.org/10.1016/j.pec.2014.12.002
2. Ong, L. M., deHaes, J. C., Hoos, A. M., & Lammes, F. B. (1995). Doctor-patients communication: A review of the literature. *Social Science & Medicine, 40*, 903–918.
3. Stewart, M. A. (1995). Effective physician-patient communication and health outcomes: A review. *Canadian Medical Association Journal, 152*(9), 1423–1433.
4. Beck, R. S., Daughtridge, R., & Sloane, P. D. (2002). Physician-patient communication in the primary care office: A systematic review. *Journal of American Board of Family Medicine, 15*, 25–38.
5. Haskard Zolnierek, K. B., & DiMatteo, M. R. (2009). Physician communication and patient adherence to treatment: a meta-analysis. *Medical Care, 47*(8), 826–834. https://doi.org/10.1097/MLR.0b013e31819a5acc

6. Ong, L. M. L., Visser, M. R. M., Lammes, F. B., & de Haes, J. C. J. M. (2000). Doctor-patient communication and cancer patients' quality of life and satisfaction. *Patient Education and Counseling, 41*(2), 145–156.

7. Vogel, B. A., Leonhart, R., & Helmes, A. W. (2009). Communication matters: the impact of communication and participation in decision making on breast cancer patients' depression and quality of life. *Patient Education and Counseling, 77*(3), 391–397.

8. Francis, V., Korsch, B. M., & Morris, M. J. (1969). *The New England Journal of Medicine, 280*, 535–540.

9. Biglu, M. H., Nateq, F., Ghojazadeh, M., & Asgharzadeh, A. (2017). Communication skills of physicians and patients' satisfaction. *Materia Socio-Medica, 29*(3), 192–195. https://doi.org/10.5455/msm.2017.29.192-195

10. Korsch, B. M., Gozzi, E. K., & Francis, V. (1968). Gaps in doctor-patient communication. *Pediatrics, 42*(5), 855–871.

11. Piette, J. D., Schillinger, D., Potter, M. B., & Heisler, M. (2003). Dimensions of patient-provider communication and diabetes self-care in an ethnically diverse population. *Journal of General Internal Medicine, 18*(8), 624–633.

12. Schillinger, D., Piette, J., Grumbach, K., et al. (2003). Closing the loop: physician communication with diabetic patients who have low health literacy. *Archives of Internal Medicine, 163*(1), 83–90. https://doi.org/10.1001/archinte.163.1.83

13. Diette, G. B., & Rand, C. (2007). The contributing role of health-care communication to health disparities for minority patients with asthma. *Chest, 132*(5), 802S–809S. https://doi.org/10.1378/chest.07-1909

14. Shen, M. J., Peterson, E. B., Costas-Muñiz, R., Hernandez, M. H., Jewell, S. T., Matsoukas, K., & Bylund, C. L. (2018). The effects of race and racial concordance on patient-physician communication: A systematic review of the literature. *Journal of Racial and Ethnic Health Disparities, 5*(1), 117–140. https://doi.org/10.1007/s40615-017-0350-4

15. Dingley, C., Daugherty, K., Derieg, M.K., et al. (2008) Improving patient safety through communication strategy enhancements. In: Henriksen, K., Battles, J.B., Keyes, M.A., et al. (eds.) *Advances in patient safety: new directions and alternative approaches* (3). : Agency for Healthcare Research and Quality.

16. Pearl, R. (2015). *Why health care is different if you're black, Latino or Poor.*

17. Appadurai, A. (1986). Ethnohistory workshop, Ethnohistory workshop, & symposium on the relationship between commodities and culture. In: *The social life of things: Commodities in cultural perspective.* Cambridge, Cambridgeshire: Cambridge University Press.

18. Manno, J. P. (2010). Commoditization and oppression. *Annals of the New York Academy of Sciences, 1185*, 164–178. https://doi.org/10.1111/j.1749-6632.2009.05285.x

19. New, C. (2001). Oppressed and oppressors? The systematic mistreatment of men. *Sociology, 35*, 729–748.

20. Lohr, K. N. (Ed.). (1990). *Medicare: A strategy for quality assurance.* National Academy Press.

21. Banaji, M. R., & Greenwald, A. G. (2013). *Blindspot: Hidden biases of good people.* Delacorte Press.

22. Cicetti, F. (2012). What is white coat syndrome? *Livestock Science.* http://www.livescience.com/36138-white-coat-syndrome-blood-pressure.html

23. DiAngelo, R. (2011). White fragility. *International Journal of Critical Pedagogy, 3*(3), 54–70.

24. Henderson, S., Horne, M., Hills, R., & Kendall, E. (2018). Cultural competence in health-care in the community: A concept analysis. *Health & Social Care in the Community, 26*(4), 590–603. https://doi.org/10.1111/hsc.12556

25. Campinha-Bacole, J., Yahle, T., & Langenkamp, M. (1996). The challenge of cultural diversity for nurse educators. *Journal of Continuing Education in Nursing, 27*(2), 59–64.

26. College of Nurses of Ontario. *Providing culturally sensitive care.* 2000. Retrieved 29 Sep 2016 from: http://www.cno.org/globalassets/docs/prac/41040_culturallysens.pdf.

27. Horton, J., & Scott, D. (2004). White students' voices in multicultural teacher education preparation. *Multicultural Education, 4*(1), 12–16.

28. McGowan, J. (2000). Multicultural teaching: African-American faculty classroom teaching experiences in predominantly white colleges and universities. *Multicultural Education, 8*(2), 19–22.
29. Whitehead, A., & Wittig, M. A. (2005). Discursive management of resistance to a multicultural education programme. *Qualitative Research in Psychology, 1*(3), 267–284.
30. Fine, M. (1997). Witnessing whiteness. In: M. Fine, L. Weis C. Powell & L. Wong (eds.), *Off white: Readings on race, power and society* (p. 57–65). : Routledge.
31. McIntosh, P. (1988). White privilege and male privilege: A personal account of coming to see correspondence through work in women's studies. In M. Anderson, & P. Hill Collins (Eds.), *Race, class and gender: An anthology* (pp. 94–105). : Wadsworth.
32. Dyer, R. (1997). *White.* Routledge.
33. Carlson, E. D., & Chamberlain, R. M. (2004). The black-white perception gap and health disparities research. *Public Health Nursing, 21*(4), 372–379.
34. Young, I. M. (1990). *Justice and the politics of difference.* Princeton University Press.
35. Scherr, C. L., Ramesh, S., Marshall-Fricker, C., & Perera, M. A. (2019). A review of African Americans' beliefs and attitudes about genomic studies: Opportunities for message design. *Frontiers in Genetics, 10*, 548. https://doi.org/10.3389/fgene.2019.00548
36. Smith, D. B. (1999). *Health care divided: Race and healing a nation.* The University of Michigan Press.
37. Byrd, W. M., & Clayton, L. A. (2000). *An American health dilemma: a medical history of African Americans and the problem of race: Belongings to 1900.* Routledge.
38. Abraham, L. K. (1993). *Mama might be better off dead: The failure of health care in urban America.* University of Chicago Press.
39. Dancy, J., & Ralston, P. A. (2002). Health promotion and black elders: Subgroups of greatest need. *Research on Aging, 24*(2), 218–242.
40. Duster, T. (2000). Forward, In F.W. Twine, & J.W. Warren (Eds.), *Racing research, researching race: Methodological dilemmas in critical race studies* (pp. xi–xiv). : New York University Press.
41. Earl, C. E., & Penney, P. J. (2001). The significance of trust in the research consent process with African Americans. *Western Journal of Nursing Research, 23*, 753–762.
42. Freedman, T. (1998). Why don't they come to pike street and ask us? Black American women's health concerns. *Social Science & Medicine, 47*, 941–947.
43. Harris, Y., Forelick, P. B., Samuels, P., & Bempong, I. (1996). Why African Americans may not be participating in clinical trials. *Journal of the National Medical Association, 88*, 630–634.
44. Mouton, C. S., Harris, S., Rovi, P., Solorzano, B. S., & Johnson, M. (1997). Barriers to black women's participation in clinical cancer trials. *Journal of the National Medical Association, 89*, 721–727.
45. Green, B. L., Partridge, E. E., Fouad, M. N., Kohler, C., Crayton, E. F., & Alexander, L. (2000). African American attitudes regarding cancer clinical trials and research studies: results from focus group methodology. *Ethnicity & Disease, 10*, 76–86.
46. Smelser, N. J., Wilson, W. J., & Mitchell, F. (Eds.). (2001). *America becoming: racial trends and their consequences (Vol. II).* National Academy Press.
47. Cose, E. (1993). *The rage of a privileged class.* Harper Perennial.
48. Carroll, R., & Shange, N. (1997). *Sugar in the raw: Voices of young black girls in America.* Three Rivers Press.
49. DuBois WEB. The souls of black folk. In: *Three negro classics.* New York: HarperCollins; 1965. p. 208–389.
50. Hooks, B. (1999). Representing whiteness in the black imagination. In R. Frankenberg (Ed.), *Displacing whiteness: Essays in social and cultural criticism.* : Duke University Press.
51. Cartwright, S. A. (1851). Report on the diseases and physical peculiarities of the negro race. *The New Orleans Medical and Surgical Journal, 7*, 691–715.

52. Pernick, M. S. (1985). *A calculus of suffering: Pain, professionalism, and anesthesia in Nineteenth-Century America*. Columbia University Press.

53. Tidyman, P. (1826). Sketch of the most remarkable diseases of the negroes of the southern states, with an account of the method of treating them, accompanied by physiological observations. *Philadelphia Journal of Medical Physics Science, 12*, 314–315.

54. Hoffman, K. M., Trawalter, S., Axt, J. R., & Oliver, M. N. (2016). Racial bias in pain assessment and treatment recommendations, and false beliefs about biological differences between blacks and whites. *Proceedings of the National Academy of Sciences, 113*(16), 4296–4301.

55. Anderson, K. O., Green, C. R., & Payne, R. (2009). Racial and ethnic disparities in pain: Causes and consequences of unequal care. *The Journal of Pain, 10*(12), 1187–1204.

56. Goyal, M. K., Kuppermann, N., Cleary, S. D., Teach, S. J., & Chamberlain, J. M. (2015). Racial disparities in pain management of children with appendicitis in emergency departments. *JAMA Pediatrics, 169*(11), 996–1002. https://doi.org/10.1001/jamapediatrics.2015.1915

57. Hoberman, J. (1997). *Darwin's athletes: how sport has damaged black America and preserved the myth of race*. Houghton Mifflin.

58. Hughey, M. (2014). Slavery, Emancipation, and the Great White Benefactor in *Django Unchained* and *Lincoln*. *Race Research Rambling*. 6 Apr. 2013. Web. 13 Dec.2014, *37*(4), 351–353.

59. Price, S. L. (1997). Is it in the genes? *Sports Illustrated, 87*, 52–55.

60. Trawalter, S., Hoffman, K. M., & Waytz, A. (2012). Racial bias in perceptions of other's pain. *PLoS ONE, 7*(11), e48546. https://doi.org/10.1371/journal.pine.0152334

61. Jayaratne, T. E., Ybarra, O., Sheldon, J. P., Brown, T. N., Feldbaum, M., Pfeffer, C. A., & Petty, E. M. (2006). White Americans' genetic lay theories of race differences and sexual orientation: Their relationship with prejudice toward blacks, and gay men and lesbians. *Group Processes & Intergroup Relations, 9*, 77–94.

62. Williams, M. J., & Eberhardt, J. L. (2008). Biological conceptions of race and the motivation to cross racial boundaries. *Journal of Personality and Social Psychology, 94*(6), 1033–1047.

63. Waytz, A., Hoffman, K. M., & Trawalter, S. (2014). A superhumanization bias in whites' perceptions of blacks. *Social Psychological and Personality Science, 6*, 352–359. https://doi.org/10.1177/1948550614553642

64. Dei, K. A. (2002). *Ties that bind: Youth & drugs in a black community*. Waveland Press, Inc.

65. Tourigny, S. (1998). Some new dying trick: African American youths "choosing" HIV/AIDS. *Qualitative Health Research, 8*, 149–167.

66. Williams, J. S., Walker, R. J., & Egede, L. E. (2016). Achieving equity in an evolving healthcare system: Opportunities and challenges. *The American Journal of the Medical Sciences, 351*(1), 33–43. https://doi.org/10.1016/j.amjms.2015.10.012

67. Institute of Medicine (US) Committee on Understanding and Eliminating Racial and Ethnic Disparities in Health Care. In B. D. Smedley, A. Y. Stith, A. R. Nelson (Eds.), *Unequal treatment: Confronting racial and ethnic disparities in health care*. : National Academies Press (US); 2003. Available from: https://www.ncbi.nlm.nih.gov/books/NBK220358/ https://doi.org/10.17226/12875.

68. Dovidio, J. E., Gaertner, S. L., Kawakami, K., & Hodson, G. (2002). Why can't we just get along? Interpersonal biases and interracial distrust. *Cultural Diversity and Ethnic Minority Psychology, 8*, 88–102.

69. Brooks, K. C. (2015). A silent curriculum. *Journal of the American Medical Association, 313*(19), 1909–1910.

70. Majumdar, B., Browne, G., Roberts, J., & Carpio, B. (2004). Effects of cultural sensitivity training on health care provider attitudes and patient outcomes. *Journal of Nursing Scholarship, 36*(2), 161–166.

71. Calvillo, E., Clark, L., Ballantyne, J. E., Pacquiao, D., Purnell, L. D., & Villarruel, A. M. (2009). Cultural competency in baccalaureate nursing education. *Journal of Transcultural Nursing, 20*, 137–145.

72. Hornborg, A. (1998). Ecosystems and world systems: accumulation as an ecological process. *Journal of World-Systems Research, 4*, 169–177.
73. Leopold, A. (1949). *A Sand County almanac: And sketches here and there.* Oxford University Press.
74. Manner, M., & Gowdy, J. (2010). The evolution of social and moral behavior: Evolutionary insights for public policy. *Ecological Economics, 69*(4), 753–761. https://doi.org/10.1016/j.ecolecon.2008.4.0121
75. Washington, H. A. (2006). *Medical apartheid: the dark history of medical experimentation on black Americans from colonial times to the present.* Doubleday.
76. Skloot, R. (2011). *The immortal life of Henrietta lacks.* Pan Books.
77. Jayawardene, S. (2015). Black mothers and C-section births: Commoditized oppression and existential violence. *Afrometrics: Research Based News.* http://wwwafrometrics.org/research-based-news/archives/09-2015
78. Plant, R. J. (2010). History of motherhood: American. In: *Encyclopedia of motherhood* (Vol. 2, pp. 507–516). Thousand Oaks, CA: SAGE Publications, Inc..
79. Morgan, J. L. (2004). *Laboring women: Reproduction and gender in New World slavery.* University of Pennsylvania Press.
80. Roberts, D. (1997). *Killing the black body: Race, reproduction, and the meaning of liberty.* Vintage Books.
81. Jones, J. (2010). *Labor of love, labor of sorrow: Black women, work, and the family from slavery to the present.* Basic Books.
82. Flavin, J. (2007). Slavery's legacy in contemporary attempts to regulate black women's reproduction. In M. Bosworth & J. Flavin (Eds.), *Race, gender, and punishment: From colonialism to the war on terror* (pp. 95–116). Rutgers University Press.
83. Ani, A. (2015). C-section and racism: "cutting" to the heart of the issue for black women and families. *Journal of African American Studies, 19*(4), 343–361.
84. Guillory, J. D. (1968). The pro-slavery arguments of Dr. Samuel a. Cartwright. *Louisiana History: The Journal of the Louisiana Historical Association, 9*, 209–227.
85. Sartin, J. S. (2004). J. Marion Sims, the father of Gynecology: Hero or villain? *Southern Medical Journal, 97*(5), 500–506.
86. Ojanuga, D. (1993). The medical ethics of the "father of gynaecology", Dr J Marion Sims. *Journal of Medical Ethics, 19*(1), 28–31.
87. Wall, L. L. (2002). Fitsari 'dan Duniya. An African (Hausa) praise song about vesicovaginal fistulas. *Obstetrics and Gynecology, 100*(6), 1328–1332.
88. Nittle, N. K. (2018). *Understanding Jim crow Laws: these regulations maintained racial apartheid in the United States.* Thought Co. Retrieved from http://www.thoughtco.com
89. Aanerud, R. (1999). Fictions of whiteness: speaking the names of whiteness in U.S. literature. In R. Frankenberg (Ed), *Displacing whiteness: Essays in social and cultural criticism* (pp. 35–39). : Duke University Press.
90. Messick D.M., Bazerman M.H., Stewart, L.. Avoiding ethical danger zones. Business Roundtable. Institute for Corporate Ethics. 2006.
91. Sabin, J. (2020). How we fail black patients in pain. Retrieved 09 Oct, 2020 from: https://www.aamc.org/news-insights/how-we-fail-black-patients-pain
92. Lown, B. A., & Manning, C. F. (2010). The Schwartz center rounds: evaluation of an interdisciplinary approach to enhancing patient-centered communication, teamwork, and provider support. *Academic Medicine, 85*(6), 1073–1081.
93. Richards, T. (1990). Chasms in communication. *British Medical Journal, 301*(6766), 1407–1408.
94. Meryn, S. (1998). Improving doctor-patient communication: not an option, but a necessity. *British Medical Journal, 316*(7149), 1922–1930.
95. Sanchez-Menegay, C., & Stalder, H. (1994). Do physicians take into account patients' expectations? *Journal of General Internal Medicine, 9*, 404–406.

96. Novack, D. H., Suchman, A. L., Clark, W., Epstein, R. M., Najberg, E., & Kaplan, C. (1997). Calibrating the physicians. Personal awareness and effective patient care. Working group on promoting physician personal awareness, American Academy on physician and patient. *Journal of the American Medical Association, 278*, 502–509.
97. Safran, D. G., Murray, A., Chang, H., Montgomery, J. E., Murphy, J., & Rogers, W. H. (2000). Linking doctor-patient relationship quality to outcomes. *Journal of General Internal Medicine, 15*(suppl), 116.
98. Levinson, W., Roter, D. L., Mullooly, J. P., Dull, V. T., & Frankel, R. M. (1997). Physician-patient communication. The relationship with malpractice claims among primary care physicians and surgeons. *Journal of the American Medical Association, 277*, 553–559.
99. Krumholz, H. M. (2013). Post-hospital syndrome-an acquired, transient condition of generalized risk. *The New England Journal of Medicine, 368*, 100–102.
100. Hafferty, F. W. (1998). Beyond curriculum reform: Confronting medicine's hidden curriculum. *Academic Medicine, 73*, 403–407.
101. Miles, S., & Leinster, S. M. (2007). Medical students' perceptions of their education environment: Expected versus actual perceptions. *Medical Education, 41*, 265–272.
102. Hammick, M., Freeth, D., Koppel, I., Reeves, S., & Barr, H. (2007). A best evidence systematic review of interporfessional education: BEME guide no. 9. *Medical Teacher, 29*, 735–751.
103. Frankenberg, R. (1993). The social construction of whiteness. In B. Rasmussen, E. Klinerberg, I. Nexica, M. Wray (Eds.), *The making and unmaking of whiteness* (pp. 72–96). : Duke University Press.
104. Johnson, H. B., & Shapiro, T. M. (2003). Good Neighborhoods, good schools: race and the "good choices" of white families. In A. W. Doane & E. Bonilla-Silva (Eds.), *White out: the continuing significance of racism* (pp. 173–187). Routledge.
105. Davis, D. A., Thomson, M. A., Oxman, A. D., & Haynes, R. B. (1995). Changing physician performance: A systematic review of the effect of continuing medical education strategies. *Journal of the American Medical Association, 274*(9), 700–705.
106. Levinson, W., & Roter, D. (1993). The effects of two continuing medical education programs on communication skills of practicing primary care physicians. *Journal of General Internal Medicine, 8*, 318–324.
107. Govere, L., & Govere, E. M. (2016). How effective is cultural competence training of healthcare providers on improving patient satisfaction of minority groups? A systematic review of literature. *Worldviews on Evidence-Based Nursing, 13*(6), 402–410. https://doi.org/10.1111/wvn.12176
108. Fraser, N. (2001). Recognition without ethics? *Theory, Culture and Society, 18*, 21–42.
109. Wachter, R. M. (2013). The experts: How to improve doctor-patient communication. *Wall Street Journal*. Retrieved from http://www.wsj.com/articles/SB10001424127887324050304578411251805908228.

B. DaNine J. Fleming, Ed.D. is an Associate Professor (tenured), Associate Chief Officer for Inclusive Excellence and Inaugural Unconscious Bias Faculty Scholar, in the Department of Diversity, Equity, and Inclusion at the Medical University of South Carolina. As a diversity and inclusion consultant, she has a passion for research and program development in the areas of leadership, social justice, civility, diversity and inclusion, ethnocultural empathy, and working with marginalized populations. She is committed to addressing the psychosocial needs of youth, children, and LGBT (lesbian, gay, bisexual, and transgender) individuals.

Part II
Characteristics of Care: Anecdotal and Scholarly Strategies for Training Professionals

Chapter 5
Appalachians and Health: The Impact of History and Culture on Healthcare Decisions and Disparities

Ava Stanzak and Rebecca Oliver-Lemieux

Complex challenges exist in Appalachian healthcare. These challenges can be difficult to address or solve without an in-depth understanding of the origin of these complexities, as well as the unique characteristics of the people who inhabit the region. Although Appalachia is a vast geographical area, within it exists regions that exhibit varying cultural beliefs and practices.

To better understand the people who inhabit the region, it is important to discuss the geography and migration that occurred to make Appalachia what it is today. Appalachia is comprised of 420 counties in 13 states—Alabama, Georgia, Kentucky, Maryland, Mississippi, New York, North Carolina, Ohio, Pennsylvania, South Caroline, Tennessee, Virginia, and West Virginia. Many of these regions are geographically isolated with 42% categorized as rural [1]. The original inhabitants of Appalachia were mostly Cherokee. European migration into these regions largely began in the eighteenth century. "The Great Migration" described by J. T. Alexander in his article "Defining the Diaspora: Appalachians in the Great Migration" emphasizes the sheer volume of individuals who migrated to the region based on financial reasons and how Appalachians were unable to make this economic transition like other immigrants who settled into the southern United States.

Mostly German and Scottish people populated the "backcountry" parts of Appalachia, other miscellaneous groups of mixed-race identity were also known to migrate, but in smaller numbers [2]. With an intermixing of various immigrants, values and attitudes toward each other clashed, which laid much of the conflict that exists in Appalachia today. The discontent from differences among the people

A. Stanzak
Primary Care, Kansas College of Osteopathic Medicine, Wichita, KS, USA

R. Oliver-Lemieux (✉)
OB/GYN, TriHealth, Cincinnati, OH, USA

migrating to the region combined with the abject poverty in Southern Appalachia, which is reported as the highest in the United States, has kept this region stagnant while other Southern regions have been able to flourish (Walls & Billings, 2009).

Healthcare Challenges in Appalachia

People in Appalachia have always cared for each other, often with no outside healthcare providers. Some of the challenges in the delivery of healthcare to Appalachia include lack of personal or public health insurance; unwillingness to travel to an unfamiliar area to receive care; delays to care as a result of trying to address the health issue through home remedies; and fear of turning loved ones over to strangers [3]. Additionally, those living in Appalachia are less likely to have health insurance and are more likely to reject government insurance.

In a study in the "Journal of Community Health" McGarvey and Leon-Verdin describe how the people of Appalachia are in poorer health than those in surrounding regions. The telephone survey revealed however unless they (Appalachians) believe they are ill, people or other habits. They also may wait longer to seek care which may lead to more serious health outcomes.

There are three major factors contributing to Appalachian health disparities: tobacco use, cancer education, and religion or faith. First, there is greater use of tobacco in Appalachia than in the rest of the United States due to community attitudes rooted in historical economic dependence on growing and trading tobacco [4]. Cigarette smoking is more common in Appalachia as is evidenced by the fact that 40% of deaths are due to chronic obstructive pulmonary disease [5]. This statistic includes deaths from Black Lung and occupational health hazards of coal mining. Environmental changes such as mountaintop removal for coal mining have impacted the citizens of Appalachia poorly, and there are few to no resources to address the outcome of these changes. Second, research indicates that people in these regions often lack facts about different types of cancer and are unaware of screening procedures [4]. Additionally, they seek answers from friends or loved ones rather than healthcare professionals about such topics, leading to further perpetuation of false information. Such lack of information and misinformation leads to high mortality and morbidity in this region.

Part of explaining areas in Appalachia can be found in theories of perceived barriers to preventative health behaviors that contend that a person's estimation of challenges or obstacles can avert positive action to address them (Glasgow, 2008). For example, children growing up with fewer resources can cause children to believe they are not able to move beyond the bounds of their socioeconomic community.

The livelihood of Appalachia has been largely dependent on the coal mining industry until now [6]. With a shift away from mining, individuals are forced to move out of this region or find new sources of income leading to perpetuation of socioeconomic barriers adversely impacting healthcare.

Impact of Appalachian Culture on Healthcare Decisions

Many of the unique cultural beliefs held by native Appalachians impact their decisions in everyday life, particularly their medical decisions. A study carried out in Southeastern Kentucky captured how those beliefs are intimately intertwined with life and death.

Palliative and hospice care are considered human right [7]; however, in many cultures, the concept of palliating pain or using hospice care at the end-of-life is both misunderstood and rejected. Cultures heavily rooted in religion and family values have alternative ways to deal with physical pain and the emotional turmoil of death; therefore, there may not be a place for palliative or hospice care in these cultures. Mostly these views persist in developing countries, but in Appalachia many of the health disparities are correlated with local values and beliefs. Developments in palliative medicine have changed the way we talk about mortality and how we approach end-of-life. The purpose of the study discussed in this portion of the chapter, was to determine if the cultural beliefs of Appalachian patients or patients' families impact their views about palliative care, and if so, is the impact positive or negative?

These data can provide insight into potential measures that can be taken to address unique disadvantages that are faced by many Appalachians. If patients of Appalachia reject palliative care or hospice based on a deeply rooted cultural belief, it is imperative that healthcare workers recognize these factors in order to provide patient-centered care. For example, rejecting an intervention due to a cultural belief that may be based on untrue facts can be addressed through education. Furthermore, these same cultural factors may be negatively or positively impacting other areas of an individual's overall well-being. Conversely, if there are Appalachian cultural values that positively impact why patients choose hospice care, it is important that these factors be acknowledged when discussing options for end-of-life with Appalachian patients.

This study took a phenomenological approach to explore the lived experiences of 30 cancer patients and their views on end-of-life. The method used for the study followed, in part, the work of Ng and von Gunten. With the authors' permission, an existing questionnaire was adapted for use in this study (Appendix A) [8]. In cooperation with the treating physician and his cancer patients at an Appalachian regional healthcare center in southeastern Kentucky 30 patient interviews were conducted. The patients were briefed by their physician during their appointment in the clinic or during rounds in the hospital before informed consent was obtained (Appendix B). Informed consent was obtained only from approved patients who could competently give written consent, and were not in acute distress. Responses were recorded manually and kept as authentic as possible throughout the transcription process. The age, sex, and diagnosis of the interviewed patients varied. They did not disclose any information about their socioeconomic status unless it emerged during a response to the questionnaire. The environment was not controlled.

Patients were seen at varying times of the day, in different locations, and at different points of their treatment. Additionally, there was no allotted time to participate in the research so interview length varied. Variation in interview responses include but are not limited to the following factors: emotional state, diagnosis, prognosis, support system, comfort level, location, time spent in the clinic or hospital that day, etc.

Some of the questions and their wording became less relevant due to a change in the location of the research from hospice center to an inpatient and outpatient cancer care center. Therefore, the distinction between use of hospice and palliative care was no longer necessary because patients were already receiving palliative care. The focus of the research shifted to use of hospice. Additionally, the reason for being seen at the facility at that time changed in relevancy because the patients were diagnosed with cancer and needed treatment; thus, they were at a cancer center to receive necessary treatment. However, knowing why the patients chose the location showed the importance of access to care in this region. Each of the patient interviews was dictated and analyzed looking for common themes.

Following the analysis, it was evident that there were four major themes impacting views on hospice and palliative care. Two of these themes strongly correlated with family values, these were grouped into familial experience and familial burden. One of the themes relied heavily on Christian values and was labeled as "God's will." The final theme involved the perception of self, which included pain and suffering as well as the wish to die with dignity.

Within these four themes, there were opposing outcomes on how these themes affected decision-making. While one or more themes were found in each patient response, the themes sometimes contributed to a positive perception of hospice/palliative care, and in other instances, the same theme contributed to negative perceptions.

Figure 5.1 demonstrates the positive or negative impact of a given theme on each patient. From the data (Fig. 5.1) it is obvious that the same theme may have caused a patient to have a positive perception of palliative or hospice care, but for a different patient, that same theme had a negative impact. Familial burden was the most prevalent theme, and familial experience being the second. Overall, the major contributor to patient values was their family, whether it was an experience a family member had with palliative or hospice care, or if it was the worry of the burden they would place on their families if they did not pursue palliative or hospice care. While it appears that God's Will did not appear as often as the others, it often appeared as a secondary theme in addition to the primary theme. Moreover, familial burden played a strong role as a secondary theme. However, pain and suffering were not seen as a secondary theme, it was only found to be the primary theme. All of the patient responses except for patient 28 strongly identified with one or more of the themes, although only one primary theme was chosen. Patient 28 was an outlier, and the response did not show a strong association with any particular opinion or belief. This patient's current situation and mental state may have impacted their ability to provide a meaningful response.

Patient Number	Familial Experience	Familial Burden	God's Will	Pain and suffering/ dying with dignity
1	+			
2	-			
3				+
4				+
5	+			
6		+		
7		+		
8	-			
9		+		
10		+		
11	-			
12		+		
13	+			
14		-		
15		+		
16	+			
17	+			
18			+	
19		+		
20				+
21	-			
22			-	
23				+
24				+
25				+
26		+		
27		+		
28				
29	+			
30		+		

Fig. 5.1 Table on themed responses by patients

Patients with prior understanding of hospice were often more articulate with their responses, whereas patients who needed an explanation of hospice tended to give shorter responses without giving the question much thought. The inability to control the environment study may have impacted the outcome due to variations in timing, recent news, treatment that day, and if they were in the clinic or hospital. Generally, those seen in the hospital were dealing with complications of a more advanced stage disease or a new diagnosis. Patients in the hospital were often significantly more talkative and receptive, depending on comfort level because they were not rushed to get to their chemotherapy treatment for that day. Due to the lack of personal information collected on patients, there was no consensus on whether there were correlations between responses and education level, socioeconomic status, past medical history, support system, etc. Additionally, the physicians had many of their own theories about patients and their beliefs, which could have been beneficial in analyzing the data. For example, the role of governmental aid in a family's decision to reject hospice care.

While in many other geographical regions in the US, the main indicator of wanting to use hospice/palliative care is pain and suffering as well as dying with dignity, in Appalachia, numerous factors affect the decreased use of palliative/hospice care. An important component of this perspective is limited access [9].

Through the analysis of the patient interviews in appendix C, there are two main factors contributing to the decision to accept or reject hospice care, both of which pertain to family. Overall, family experience contributed most significantly to the rejection of hospice care, while family burden contributed most positively. This data suggests that Appalachian patient identity is intertwined with family, and belief of personal outcomes are like those of their loved ones thus decisions are based largely on family experience.

For some patients, news of a bad CT image or addition of chemo treatments affected their outlook and impacted their responses. A second or third interview would have eliminated bias; however, these factors cannot be ignored because those working in end-of-life care must consider emotional state when comprehending decisions and to what extent emotional turmoil may interfere with the ability to consent.

The findings in this small but insightful study suggest that there are prevalent cultural factors impacting Appalachian patients in making decisions about end-of-life that extend beyond access to care. The concept of end-of-life care encompasses all aspects of the patient's life thus knowing these factors allows caregivers to care for their patient's emotional, mental, spiritual, and physical well-being. It is apparent that these factors impact decision-making about palliative/hospice care acceptance or rejection, and most likely impact their decision-making in other aspects of their overall health. This enables public health initiatives to be tailored to this population.

Addressing Healthcare Issues

Religious and community organizations have attempted to address the issue of healthcare delivery in Appalachia with success. Not all regions have been reached but the attempt can be noted by the fact that Jeff Eastman, CEO of Remote Area Medical (RAM) stated in a CNN interview in October 2019 that they had treated over 750,000 individuals since their establishment.

Smaller faith-based free clinics can be found in many cities and towns across Appalachia. Some use recreational vehicles that have been outfitted for a clinic and take the healthcare to the patients. These mobile clinics have routine stops and a schedule, so people know when and where they can be seen for healthcare.

These organizations are successful for a few reasons: services are free of charge or based on income, the providers are from Appalachia or regions with the same value system, and patients do not have to travel far from their homes to seek care. If a higher level of care is needed or hospitalization, arrangements are made by the organizations providing the care to have the patient cared for by someone close to home. In some areas, medical specialists travel to the communities on a schedule that can be accessed by primary care providers. When people see specialists in their own community, they are more likely to keep the appointment and have an improved outcome. Some Appalachian communities have free (or inexpensive) transportation available for people so they can get to healthcare facilities within the community. These services are funded by the local town or by the state government. In most cases, they are an afterthought and if money runs out, the services either have decreased availability or cease. Services may be available, but the people are not aware of or fear the expense. It may take years for these services to be arranged in a community, especially if funds are not readily available. There is also the issue of maintaining vehicles, insurance, getting drivers, and housing the services.

Currently, healthcare in Appalachia is being addressed using free clinics and home visits by the free clinic system. As previously mentioned, a lack of cultural competence on the part of healthcare providers can be a barrier to seeking care. Inability to understand the dialect and lack of awareness regarding the culture can alienate Appalachian communities. Healthcare providers who plan to work in Appalachia should invest in researching the culture, economics, and dialect of the areas. Once people have a difficult experience with a healthcare provider, they are much less likely to return for care, even if it is emergent. Patience, excellent listening skills, and empathy are crucial for success. Allowing medical students, residents, nursing, and physician assistant students to have part of their training take place in Appalachia may help them decide if the area is a good fit for future employment.

In the last 25 years, several new osteopathic medical schools have been initiated in Appalachia with the sole intent of producing more healthcare providers for the area [10]. These schools are not only graduating physicians but physician's assistants and nurse practitioners. Most of these students are completing their education in rural areas, and recruitment at these institutions places an emphasis on recruiting from rural Appalachia. There are few scholarships for these students, so they rely heavily on student loans. A program that created a subsidy for these rural students would allow them to remain in Appalachia and care for their own communities. Subsidies should not reflect as income and should not impact physician salaries.

Where medical students train is where many remain to practice. Creating more postgraduate training programs in Appalachia would be beneficial in keeping physicians in their own community. Residency programs have a government-imposed "cap" on the number of residents in a program based on the population of the area. Removing this limit in underserved regions would help with the shortage. Keeping rural people together for healthcare would result in patient compliance, continuity, and overall better access to healthcare services.

To meet the challenges of healthcare needs in Appalachia, a subsidy is necessary to help healthcare providers and healthcare facilities continue to provide services to Appalachian patients. This subsidy might be loan forgiveness for physicians and other healthcare providers for the time spent working in the area. Allowing healthcare facilities to accept any insurance and waiving a copay may also help with patient care. Education of patients regarding health insurance and Medicaid may help people obtain the resources needed for adequate healthcare.

To obtain more healthcare providers in Appalachia, some states have created a partnership between medical schools in the state and underserved areas searching for more providers. These organizations contact the alumni associations at medical schools, and work together with the school's database to see what specialties former students pursue. Interested resident physicians are offered a subsidy while still in training, to go to an underserved area to practice when their residency is completed. This subsidy is considered a loan and is forgiven if the physician remains in the area for a specified length of time. Some of these programs also recruit nurse practitioners, physician assistants, and dentists. The Tennessee Rural Partnership has achieved this over the past 10 years and has helped recruit over 100 practitioners to help rural and underserved communities in the state of Tennessee. This program allows healthcare providers to return to their community to practice without the fear of financial insecurity.

The Tobacco Region Revitalization Commission has provided grant money in Virginia to create new healthcare programs and help providers sustain a practice in rural areas of the state [11]. This program, and those like it, require a grant for planned services. This is a deterrent to many, as grant writing is tedious, must be exact, and few healthcare providers are proficient in these skills. Grant writers usually need to be paid thus presenting another challenge. Grant processing can take months to years, so the delay may decrease interest in the project. The organization may not get the grant and must search for resources again.

This process must be easier for healthcare providers to access, have reciprocity in all states, and look at individual resources in communities when granting money.

The Appalachia Regional Commission has worked for years to create programs that help the people of Appalachia, these programs include child abuse prevention, recruiting and retaining nurses, having physician assistant students and medical students train in these communities, and create post-graduate medical training programs at some of the hospitals in the area.

Some of the strategies used by the Appalachia Regional Commission include:

– Using best practices to develop targeted approaches to wellness and disease prevention.
– To create partnerships to educate children and families about health risks.
– Using telecommunication to reduce healthcare costs (may be problematic due to lack of phone service in some areas).
– Encourage development and expansion of health professions education services in the area.

Things that are working currently to address some of the above issues is the aforementioned free clinic model. Having a healthcare team go directly to the population works if there is a set schedule and if the hours can accommodate the population, such as hours that accommodate work schedule. Health fairs such as Remote Area Medical, mentioned above, have schedules a year in advance and some people travel across several states to get care. Not everyone can be seen at every event, and there is difficulty in securing follow-up. Local health fairs can identify health problems in their community but must plan to provide some sort of follow-up care to be effective in helping people.

Providers can arrange to make home visits to people who may not have reliable transportation, or who have a disability that prevents them from traveling. Home visits are a billable service by most insurance plans including Medicare and Medicaid. Setting up regular clinics at schools and churches can work well. Having a clinic recreational vehicle is also an excellent way to take healthcare to the population. The challenge in this is to have the financial resources to provide the staff, supplies, and a location for clinics. Most of these types of clinics have relied on donations and volunteer services to provide services. This causes limitation of services which causes limited participation by potential patients. Continuity of care is a problem when healthcare providers change constantly and there is no scheduled time for follow-up care.

The problems existing within the healthcare systems in Appalachia cannot be solved quickly or with one simple solution. The problems are multifactorial and complex. Recruiting more healthcare providers, more clinic facilities, and better education for the Appalachian population will take financial resources. Large healthcare systems (corporate medicine) must allow employed healthcare providers to provide these services regularly in needy areas.

Money must be accessible after completion of a needs assessment that is uncomplicated and user-friendly. The money must be awarded quickly so results are seen quickly. Having a lengthy, inefficient process that involves people not within the community has a negative impact on the process and the outcome. This encourages the culture of "getting by" and futility seen in Appalachia for the last 100 years.

Caring for the health of the people of Appalachia will require money, expedited program access, and culturally competent healthcare providers who have trained in the area and can afford to work and live within their community. This will be the ultimate multidisciplinary effort between the local and federal government, medical educational facilities, and individuals who want to care for their community. Cost sharing and streamlined evaluation of needs will be instrumental in achieving accessible healthcare for the people of Appalachia.

References

1. Griffith, B. N., et al. (2011). Self-rated health in rural Appalachia: Health perceptions are incongruent with health status and health behaviors. *BMC Public Health, 11*(1), 1–8.
2. Drake, R. B. (2001). The road to poverty: The making of wealth and hardship in Appalachia. *The Journal of American History, 87*(4), 1477.
3. McGarvey, E. L., et al. (2011). Health disparities between Appalachian and non-Appalachian counties in Virginia USA. *Journal of Community Health, 36*(3), 348–356.
4. Behringer, B., & Friedell, G. H. (2006). Appalachia: Where place matters in health. *Preventing Chronic Disease, 3*, 4.
5. Hendryx, M., Ahern, M. M., & Nurkiewicz, T. R. (2007). Hospitalization patterns associated with Appalachian coal mining. *Journal of Toxicology and Environmental Health, Part A, 70*(24), 2064–2070.
6. Betz, M. R., et al. (2015). Coal mining, economic development, and the natural resources curse. *Energy Economics, 50*, 105–116.
7. Brennan, F. (2007). Palliative care as an international human right. *Journal of Pain and Symptom Management, 33*(5), 494–499.
8. Ng, K., & von Gunten, C. F. (1998). Symptoms and attitudes of 100 consecutive patients admitted to an acute hospice/palliative care unit. *Journal of Pain and Symptom Management, 16*(5), 307–316.
9. Cai, Y., & Lalani, N. (2022). Examining barriers and facilitators to palliative care access in rural areas: a scoping review. *The American Journal of Hospice & Palliative Care, 39*(1), 123–130.
10. Casto, J. E. (2001). A medical school for the mountains: training doctors for rural care. *Appalachia, 34*(3), 24–29.
11. Developing a Diverse Economy in Southern and Southwest Virginia. Virginia Tobacco Region Revitalization Commission, https://www.revitalizeva.org/.

Ava Stanzck, D.O. is a licensed Pediatrician who has served patients in Tennessee and Texas as a primary care physician and a clinical director in an academic college of medicine. She has also served as a member of the National Board of Osteopathic Medical Examiners for many years.

Rebecca Oliver-Lemieux, D.O., M.B.E. is a resident in obstetrics/gynecology at Tri Health, Cincinnati, Ohio. She received her education at U Pike-Kentucky College of Osteopathic Medicine and has conducted research in ethics and hospice care. Dr. Oliver was a research assistant while completing her medical education.

Chapter 6
A Culture of Stigmatization: The Healthcare of Minoritized Populations

Asia T. McCleary-Gaddy and Drexler James

Introduction

As healthcare and academic professionals examine innovative pathways to improve patient health, research reveals that while medical care (e.g., access to care, quality of care) contributes 10–15% to premature death in the United States, socioeconomic conditions (e.g., income, debt, education) contributes an estimated 60% [1]. The aforementioned "conditions" in which people are born, grow, live, work, and age are known as the social determinants of health (SDOH; [2]). SDOH are broad and include income, education, housing, food security, employment, social support, identity facets, racism, and discrimination. SDOH are shaped by the distribution of money, power, and resources at global, national, and local levels [2].

Prior research has demonstrated that SDOH are major predictors of adverse health outcomes, including infant mortality, diabetes, hypertension, obesity, length, and quality of life [3–6]. Given that these SDOH are oftentimes preventable, healthcare professionals use evidence-based approaches to examine the effects (mediating and moderating) of SDOH on health. In addition, through a SDOH curriculum, health professional students learn more about the pervasiveness of health inequities that are more likely to affect individuals who *systematically* experience greater social or economic obstacles as a result of one or more stigmatized identities.

A. T. McCleary-Gaddy (✉)
Psychiatry and Behavioral Sciences, McGovern Medical School at the University of Texas
Health Science Center at Houston, Houston, TX, USA
e-mail: Asia.t.mcclearygadddy@uth.tmc.edu

D. James
Assistant Professor of Psychology, Univeristy of Minnesota, Twin Cities, Minneapolis, MN, USA

Stigma: A Social Determinant of Health

According to sociologist Erving Goffman [7] "stigma is an attribute that extensively discredits an individual, reducing him or her from a whole and usual person to a tainted, discounted one." (p. 3) Stigmatizing attributes may be visible (e.g., an individual who is obese) or invisible (e.g., an individual who has a mental illness), perceived to be controllable (e.g., HIV/AIDS) or uncontrollable (e.g., sexual orientation), and linked to appearance (e.g., a physical deformity), behavior (e.g., drug use), or group membership (e.g., African American). Crocker, Major, and Steele [8] suggest that stigmatization occurs when a person is "perceived to possess some attribute or characteristic that conveys a social identity that is devalued in a particular social context" (p. 505). Thus, people who are stigmatized are believed to have an attribute that leads to devalued identity(ies).

Stigma exists on three interrelated levels: intrapersonal, interpersonal, and structural [9]. *Intrapersonal stigma* refers to the psychological processes in which individuals engage in response to stigma such as self-stigma: the internalization of negative societal views about your group. In contrast, *interpersonal stigma* refers to interactions that occur between the stigmatized and the non-stigmatized such as attitudes of prejudice and discriminatory behaviors. Last, *structural stigma* refers to stigma at the macrolevel. Structural stigma is defined as the economic and political pressures on a culture that produce social and institutional policies that limit opportunities for the stigmatized group [10]. Structural stigma includes institutional policies that intentionally constrain the opportunities of people with stigmatized identities but also unintentional policies whose consequences impede the options of stigmatized groups. Therefore, in a more comprehensive conceptualization, stigmatization is defined as the co-occurrence of labeling, stereotyping, separation, status loss, and discrimination in a context in which power is exercised [9].

Overview

Hatzenbuehler and colleagues [11] argue that all stigma-related dynamics have a significant effect on individual and population health comparable to the other social determinants of health. Researchers also estimate that stigma in a healthcare context contributes to more disparity in life expectancy than stigma in the general population [12]. Various models of stigma argue that interpersonal, structural, and intrapersonal levels of stigma individually and interactively contribute to poor health outcomes, especially among minoritized populations (see [13]). For example, the *biopsychosocial model of racism* [14] argues that race stigma (i.e., racism) is a chronic stressor for racial/ethnic minorities that, once experienced, leads to various psychological and physiological stress responses. Similarly, the *Internalized Stigma Model* (IMS) of mental illness suggests that both interpersonal and intrapersonal forms of stigma of mental illness reduce self-esteem and help-seeking behaviors among those with mental illness [15]. In particular, the IMS suggests that awareness of public stigma can lead to its internalization as self-stigma, which then decreases self-esteem and intentions to seek psychological help [15].

Other models focus on how stigmatization in healthcare settings can lead also contribute to minority-majority health disparities. For example, Knaak and Patten's [16] model suggests that stigma manifests in several different ways in healthcare settings, including a lack of or limited diversity-related healthcare training and healthcare provider-held anti-minority stigmas. As an example, results from a systematic review by Van Boekel et al. [17] found that health professionals generally had negative attitudes toward patients with substance use disorders, which affect their treatment of these patients. In addition, they found that health professionals also lacked adequate education, training, and support structures in working with this patient group, altogether contributing to suboptimal health care for patients with substance use disorders.

To contribute to this literature, this chapter reviews scholarship examining the health consequences of stigma among minoritized populations—populations of people who have less power than their peers. Here we provide evidence of the pervasiveness of stigma within healthcare and the pernicious consequences of stigma on overall health. First, using some examples, we highlight the current research on stigma and health of multiple communities including: (1) racial and ethnic minorities, (2) gender and sexual minorities, (3) individuals living with mental illness, and (4) individuals who are overweight. Following, we discuss areas of future research, methods to cope with and combat stigma, and the implications for health professional education and practice.

Stigma and Minoritized Populations

Weight Stigma

Weight stigma is defined as the social devaluation and denigration of people perceived to carry excess weight and leads to prejudice, negative stereotyping, and discrimination toward those people [18]. Weight stigma is relatively under-studied compared to other forms of stigma (e.g., race, gender), although it is reported to be more common, severe, and socially acceptable [19, 20]. This is especially troubling given that around two-thirds of Americans are either overweight or obese [21]. In the healthcare setting, overweight and obese patients are susceptible to weight stigma from physicians, nurses, medical students, and dental students [22].

For example, Hebl and Xu [23] found that primary care physicians reported that seeing obese patients was a greater waste of their time and that heavier patients were more annoying than patients with lower body weights. Physicians also reported having less patience and desire to help patients who were overweight/obese. Medical students also express that obese patients are more difficult to work with [24]. In the same way, research shows that nurses also hold largely negative weight-based attitudes toward patients who are overweight/obese, including these patients being lazy, lacking in self-control, and noncompliant [25]. Last, about 30% of dental students report that their obese patients are lazier than non-obese patients and about 17% reported that it was difficult for them to feel empathy for an obese patient [26].

Researchers interested in the obesity epidemic have identified chronic stress as a potential mechanism through which stigma and stigmatizing environments increase the risk for negative health outcomes [27]. Tomiyama [28] outlined the Cyclic Obesity/Weight-based Stigma (COBWEBS) model that depicts weight stigma as a positive feedback loop wherein weight stigma catalyzes weight gain through increased eating and other biobehavioral mechanisms. The COBWEBS model first characterizes weight stigma as a psychological stressor. The stress induced by weight stigma initiates emotional responses such as intense feelings of shame, physiological responses such as an increase in the stress hormone cortisol, and behavioral responses such as "comfort eating." As a result, weight increases weight gain in overweight individuals, which increases their susceptibility to weight stigma.

Much research on weight stigma has focused on the role of the hormone *cortisol*. Cortisol, a stress-related hormone, promotes fat storage and eating behavior [29]. A typical response to a stressor is characterized by a sharp increase in cortisol followed by a slow decline. However, McCleary-Gaddy and colleagues [30] found that overweight individuals who are placed in a weight-stigmatizing situation exhibit a blunted cortisol response. That is, their cortisol response is characterized by relatively small fluctuations following a stressor. Other studies document that people who experience childhood victimization or racial discrimination have blunted cortisol responses to acute stressors [31, 32]. Blunted cortisol responsivity is especially important to individuals who are overweight as cortisol plays an important role in the distribution of adipose tissue, which is implicated in cardiovascular disease and type 2 diabetes [28].

Mental Health Stigma

Mental health stigma refers to the devalued social identity one may possess due to the negative attribute of mental illness [33]. One of the most commonly cited sources of stigma for people with mental illness is the structural stigma within the healthcare system [34]. This is concerning as about one in five US adults lives with a mental illness [35].

Schulze [36] discusses how legislative policies create a low quality of services for people with mental illness, complications for accessing treatment, forceful approaches to care, and inadequate funding of mental health research and services

[34]. In a review of nearly 1000 mental health-related proposed bills in 2002, researchers found 1% were discriminatory (e.g., restricted placement of mental health facilities) and 4% reduced privacy (e.g., permitting disclosure of mental health information in certain circumstances; [37]). Other work also shows that physicians are less likely to accept insurance coverage for some mental health services because of the low monetary reimbursement [38], which exacerbates physician shortage and low quality of services within the mental healthcare domain [39].

Mental illness stigma also has inward-facing impacts on health professionals' own willingness to seek help or disclose mental health problems [40]. Research has found that dentists experience greater levels of anxiety and depressive disorders as a result of the stress of their occupation, but are less likely to seek help because of self-stigma [41]. Nurses who suffer from mental illness often felt that they were targets for exclusionary behaviors including shunning reactions from supervisors and expulsion from the workplace [42]. However, Arvaniti and colleagues [43] found that nurses report the least favorable attitude toward people with mental illness when compared to doctors, medical students, and other healthcare personnel. For medical students and physicians, mental illness stigma elicits perceptions of incompetence and creates stagnation in career trajectory in the competitive medical setting. For example, Hampton [44] found that the most frequently cited barriers to treatment were lack of confidentiality (37%), stigma (30%), and fear of documentation on academic record (24%). Since mental illness is a concealable stigma, an identity people can choose to make known to others, many healthcare professionals may never reveal the status of their mental health, which may increase the risk of suicidal behaviors, depression, anxiety, and exacerbate the mental illness [44].

Racial/Ethnic Minority Stigma

US racial minorities have a shorter life expectancy and poorer physical and mental health than their US non-Hispanic White counterparts [45]. Previous and extensive work shows that race-related stigma, that is racism, is a significant cause of these health disparities [46, 47]. Models of racism (e.g., biopsychosocial model of racism; [14]; multidimensional conceptualization of racism-related stress; [48]) suggest that racism is a stressor that can result in psychological/physiological damage among racial/ethnic minorities (also see [49]). For example, among racial/ethnic minorities experiences with racial discrimination increases the body's physiological stress responses, including increased blood pressure and heart rate [50] and increased cortisol production (for meta-analysis see [51]).

Within the healthcare domain, race stigma influences healthcare providers' attitudes and interactions with racial/ethnic minority patients. For example, Van Ryn and Burke [52] found that physicians were more likely to rate their Black/African American as less intelligent and less likely to adhere to treatment regimens. Van

Ryn and Burke [52] suggest that these negative racial attitudes might account for racial/ethnic disparities in the quality of healthcare [53], treatment recommendations [54], patient–physician relationships [55], and treatment recovery [56], where racial/ethnic minorities experience oftentimes experience poorer outcomes than their White counterparts. Indeed, racial/ethnic minorities are less likely to seek professional healthcare for fear of experiencing racial discrimination by their healthcare provider [57]. Other work suggests that this perceived racial bias also increases racial/ethnic minority patients' mistrust of their healthcare provider, which can lead to poor medication adherence [58].

Experiences with racial/ethnic discrimination can also lead racial/ethnic minorities to internalize race-related stigma, that is, *internalized racism*. Internalized racism (IR) is a form of racism that leads people to internalize beliefs and stereotypes about their race/ethnicity [59]. Internalized racism is associated with poor physical (e.g., systolic blood pressure; [60]) and mental (e.g., depression; [61]) health outcomes. Indeed, a recent meta-analysis found that internalized racism (IR) was associated with poorer mental and physical health outcomes among RE minorities [62]. This increased risk of poorer health might also result from a decreased willingness to seek healthcare resulting from increased internalized racism [63]. Other work shows that internalized racism exacerbates the negative health effects of experiencing discrimination. For example, Chae et al. [64] found that among Black/African American men with high levels of internalized racism, experiencing discrimination was associated with shorter leukocyte telomere length (LTL) while for those with low internalized racism, experiencing discrimination was associated with lower LTL.

LGBTQ+ Stigma

Sexual minorities (i.e., those who identify as non-heterosexual) report poorer health relative to heterosexuals including higher rates of substance use and abuse [65], cardiovascular disease [66], and suicidality [67]. In a national sample of American adults, Rice and colleagues (2019) found that sexual minority participants reported higher rates of general discrimination, victimization, and healthcare discrimination than heterosexual adults. Indeed, Meyer [68] posited the "sexual minority stress" model to explain how experienced sexual minority stigma (e.g., discrimination, internalized homophobia) increases sexual minorities' risks of poor health outcomes. Previous research shows that experienced stigma is positively associated with poor mental [69], physical [70], and sexual health [71] outcomes among sexual minorities.

Other research has focused specifically on the ways in which stigma affects sexual minorities within the healthcare context. For example, in a sample of African American sexual minority women, Li et al. [72] found that 46.2% of participants reported negative healthcare experience within the past 5 years due to their sexual orientation. Li et al. [72] also found that increased experiences with healthcare discrimination predicted reduced healthcare service utilization. In the same way, Steele et al. [73] found that bisexual women were likely to report an unmet need for mental healthcare as cisgender heterosexual women. Here the authors argue that in addition to interpersonal stigma experienced by healthcare professionals the systemic exclusion of sexual minorities from healthcare systems also contributes to sexual minority health disparities.

In fact, in a sample of 180 physicians Jabson et al. [74] found that 171 (95%) of physicians reported that they were aware, and 9 (5%) were unaware, that patients in their practice identified as gay, lesbian, or bisexual, and 171 (95%) reported that they were aware, and 9 (5%) were unaware, that patients in their practice identified as transgender. However, despite this awareness, the sample of physicians still held overall negative attitudes about sexual minority patients. Citing the importance of structural-level policies at hospitals, Jabson et al. [74] found that physicians at a hospital with Healthcare Equality Index (HEI) training/policies held less negative attitudes toward sexual minorities than those at a hospital without HEI training/policies. These physician-held biases have consequences for patient treatment. For example, Calabrese et al. [75] found that greater explicit bias against gay men is linked to provider decisions among medical students, such as less willingness to prescribe Pre-Exposure Prophylaxis (PrEP), a drug that reduces HIV risk.

Future Research Considerations for Stigma and Health

Intersectional Stigma

Oftentimes, stigma is examined along one identity dimension (e.g., race) rather than along multiple identity dimensions (e.g., race and gender). To address the limitations of such investigations, especially in relation to health and well-being, Turan et al. [76] reintroduced "intersectional stigma": a concept that characterizes the convergence of multiple stigmatized identities within a person or group. An intersectional perspective allows health professionals to think holistically about how living with multiple stigmatized identities affects behaviors, as well as individual and population health. For example, socioeconomic status (SES), whether measured by income, education, or occupational status, is among the most robust determinants of variations in health outcomes throughout the world [77]. Understanding the complex ways in which stigmatized identities such as race/ethnicity, gender, sexual orientation, and SES uniquely and in combination, influence health outcomes is a critical task in addressing disparities across the socioeconomic spectrum [78].

Intersectional stigma has been repeatedly associated with worse health behaviors and outcomes. For example, Eisner and researchers [79] found that African Americans were associated with greater disease severity and greater risk of acute COPD, but these differences no longer persisted after controlling for SES variables. In another study investigating transgender individuals, researchers found higher levels of violence was reported for transgender youth who were low income [80]. Collectively, this suggests that lower SES exacerbates the health outcomes for individuals who already possess one stigmatized identity.

Future research should aim to understand the ways in which childhood SES and other stigmatized identities contribute to adult health inequities, including the psychosocial and physiological pathways [76]. Research that investigates a single health-related stigma without including the co-experience of other stigmas is likely to have limited success in reducing health inequities because it does not accurately reflect the lived experiences of our society [76].

Racial Stigma and White American Health

Research examining racial stigma and its relationship to health and mortality overwhelmingly examine these relationships among racial/ethnic minority populations. However, recent scholarly works suggest that racial stigma (structural, interpersonal, and internalized) can lead to poor health among non-Hispanic White Americans in the US, that is, the racial majority. Recently, Williams et al. [81] highlighted a need for research that examines how racism effects the health of non-Hispanic whites in the US. Indeed, similar to the negative health effects of racism on minority health, research shows that self-reported experiences of discrimination are also associated with poorer health outcomes among US whites. For example, Mustillo et al. [82] found that self-reported experiences of racial discrimination were associated with higher rates of both preterm births and low birth weight babies in a sample of 352 African American and White American women. Similarly, Tomfohr et al. [83] found that higher endorsement of everyday discrimination was associated with less diastolic blood pressure (DBP) and systolic blood pressure (SBP) dipping among Black and White American men and women.

In the same way, scholars (e.g., [59]) argue that White Americans' internalization of racism—the internalization, among members of a dominant, privileged, or powerful racial/ethnic groups, of attitudes, beliefs or ideologies about the inferiority of other racial/ethnic groups and/or the superiority of their own racial/ethnic group—can also have negative health consequences for them. Internalization of such beliefs can lead White Americans to espouse beliefs that can, directly and indirectly, affect their health. As an example, Tesler [84] found that anti-Black racial resentment was associated with increased opposition to the Affordable Care Act (ACA) by White Americans. Replicating these findings, Metzl [85] found, in interviews, that lower income White men report that even to risk to their own health that they would not vote for policies that would give racial/ethnic minority groups or immigrants more access to healthcare (e.g., the ACA). Here, we see that some racial majority members will risk their own life and health to maintain the racial hierarchy. This is particularly telling as Metzl [85] shows that states that introduced the ACA saw a reduction in overall mortality of 6.1% from 2011 to 2015.

Conclusion

Despite a growing understanding of the importance of SDH, the inclusion of this material into standard training curricula remains sporadic, and when it is included, it is often considered optional [86]. As the field of healthcare transitions into a physician advocacy model, it is important that we embed research on the pervasiveness of stigma into the curriculum. Health professionals would benefit from a social science curriculum that details how the thoughts, feelings, and behaviors of individuals are influenced by the actual, imagined, and implied presence of others (e.g., social psychology; [87]).

Specifically, discussing stigma as a social determinant of health addresses three levels of how an individual is affected. It also promotes greater self-reflection of our healthcare professionals with the goal of better healthcare for all. These discussions may also act as a catalyst for a greater conversation about inclusive coping mechanisms. For example, coping mechanisms associated with weight stigma can range from harmful (e.g., maladaptive eating behaviors) to beneficial (e.g., healthy lifestyle change; [88]). Greater knowledge of culturally sensitive coping mechanisms as a response to stigma can also increase healthcare for all. Last, while this chapter was not intended to be comprehensive of all stigma faced by the various minoritized communities, it provides a broad overview of how stigma contributes to ill-health among minoritized populations. In particular, this chapter serves to demonstrate, briefly, how stigma (structural, interpersonal, and internalized) affects healthcare service, particularly for patients who are members of minoritized populations in the US.

References

1. Schroeder, S. A. (2007). We can do better—improving the health of the American people. *The New England Journal of Medicine, 357*(12), 1221–1228.
2. WHO (World Health Organization). What are the social determinants of health? 2020. Available from: http://www.who.int/social_determinants/sdh_definition/en/. Accessed 8 Oct 2020
3. Chetty, R., Stepner, M., Abraham, S., Lin, S., Scuderi, B., Turner, N., Cutler, D., et al. (2016). The association between income and life expectancy in the United States, 2001-2014. *JAMA, 315*(16), 1750–1766.
4. Kim, D., & Saada, A. (2013). The social determinants of infant mortality and birth outcomes in Western developed nations: A cross-country systematic review. *International Journal of Environmental Research and Public Health, 10*(6), 2296–2335.
5. Kreatsoulas, C., & Anand, S. S. (2010). The impact of social determinants on cardiovascular disease. *The Canadian Journal of Cardiology, 26*, 8C–13C.
6. Reidpath, D. D., Burns, C., Garrard, J., Mahoney, M., & Townsend, M. (2002). An ecological study of the relationship between social and environmental determinants of obesity. *Health & Place, 8*(2), 141–145.
7. Goffman, E. (1963). *Stigma: Notes on the Management of Spoiled Identity*. Prentice Hall.
8. Crocker, J., Major, B., & Steele, C. M. (1998). Social stigma. In D. Gilbert, S. T. Fiske, & G. Lindzey (Eds.), *Handbook of social psychology* (Vol. 2, 4th ed., pp. 504–553). McGraw-Hill.

9. Link, B. G., & Phelan, J. C. (2001). Conceptualizing stigma. *Annual review of. Social Forces,* *27*(1), 363–385.

10. Hatzenbuehler, M. L. (2016). Structural stigma: Research evidence and implications for psychological science. *The American Psychologist, 71*(8), 742–751. https://doi.org/10.1037/amp0000068

11. Hatzenbuehler, M. L., Phelan, J. C., & Link, B. G. (2013). Stigma as a fundamental cause of population health inequalities. *American Journal of Public Health, 103*(5), 813–821. https://doi.org/10.2105/AJPH.2012.301069

12. Henderson, C., Noblett, J., Parke, H., Clement, S., Caffrey, A., Gale-Grant, O., Thornicroft, G., et al. (2014). Mental health-related stigma in health care and mental health-care settings. *Lancet Psychiatry, 1*(6), 467–482.

13. Eccleston, C. P. (2008). The psychological and physical health effects of stigma: The role of self-threats. *Social and Personality Psychology Compass, 2*(3), 1345–1361.

14. Clark, R., Anderson, N. B., Clark, V. R., & Williams, D. R. (2013). *Racism as a stressor for African Americans: A biopsychosocial model* (pp. 79–103). Jossey-Bass/Wiley.

15. Lannin, D. G., Vogel, D. L., Brenner, R. E., & Tucker, J. R. (2015). Predicting self-esteem and intentions to seek counseling: The internalized stigma model. *The Counseling Psychologist, 43*(1), 64–93.

16. Knaak, S., & Patten, S. (2016). A grounded theory model for reducing stigma in health professionals in Canada. *Acta Psychiatrica Scandinavica, 134*, 53–62.

17. Van Boekel, L. C., Brouwers, E. P., Van Weeghel, J., & Garretsen, H. F. (2013). Stigma among health professionals towards patients with substance use disorders and its consequences for healthcare delivery: Systematic review. *Drug and Alcohol Dependence, 131*(1–2), 23–35.

18. Tomiyama, A. J. (2014). Weight stigma is stressful. A review of evidence for the cyclic obesity/weight-based stigma model. *Appetite, 82*, 8–15.

19. Brochu, P. M., & Esses, V. M. (2011). What's in a name? The effects of the labels "fat" versus "overweight" on weight bias 1. *Journal of Applied Social Psychology, 41*(8), 1981–2008.

20. Puhl, R. M., & Heuer, C. A. (2009). The stigma of obesity: A review and update. *Obesity, 17*(5), 941.

21. Ogden, C. L., Carroll, M. D., Kit, B. K., & Flegal, K. M. (2014). Prevalence of childhood and adult obesity in the United States, 2011-2012. *JAMA, 311*(8), 806–814.

22. Puhl, R., & Brownell, K. D. (2001). Bias, discrimination, and obesity. *Obesity Research, 9*(12), 788–805.

23. Hebl, M. R., & Xu, J. (2001). Weighing the care: Physicians' reactions to the size of a patient. *International Journal of Obesity, 25*(8), 1246–1252.

24. Wear, D., Aultman, J. M., Varley, J. D., & Zarconi, J. (2006). Making fun of patients: Medical students' perceptions and use of derogatory and cynical humor in clinical settings. *Academic Medicine, 81*(5), 454–462.

25. Brown, I. (2006). Nurses' attitudes towards adult patients who are obese: Literature review. *Journal of Advanced Nursing, 53*(2), 221–232.

26. Magliocca, K. R., Jabero, M. F., Alto, D. L., & Magliocca, J. F. (2005). Knowledge, beliefs, and attitudes of dental and dental hygiene students toward obesity. *Journal of Dental Education, 69*(12), 1332–1339.

27. McCleary-Gaddy, A. T., Miller, C. T., Grover, K. W., Hodge, J. J., & Major, B. (2019). Weight stigma and hypothalamic-pituitary-adrenocortical Axis reactivity in individuals who are overweight. *Annals of Behavioral Medicine, 53*(4), 392–398. https://doi.org/10.1093/abm/kay042

28. Tomiyama, A. J., Epel, E. S., McClatchey, T. M., Poelke, G., Kemeny, M. E., McCoy, S. K., & Daubenmier, J. (2014). Associations of weight stigma with cortisol and oxidative stress independent of adiposity. *Health Psychology, 33*(8), 862.

29. Himmelstein, M. S., Incollingo Belsky, A. C., & Tomiyama, A. J. (2015). The weight of stigma: Cortisol reactivity to manipulated weight stigma. *Obesity, 23*(2), 368–374.

30. McCleary-Gaddy, A. T., & Miller, C. T. (2019). Negative religious coping as a mediator between perceived prejudice and psychological distress among African Americans: A structural equation modeling approach. *Psychology of Religion and Spirituality, 11*(3), 257–265. https://doi.org/10.1037/rel0000228
31. Bevans, K., Cerbone, A., & Overstreet, S. (2008). Relations between recurrent trauma exposure and recent life stress and salivary cortisol among children. *Development and Psychopathology, 20*(1), 257–272.
32. Richman, L. S., & Jonassaint, C. (2008). The effects of race-related stress on cortisol reactivity in the laboratory: Implications of the Duke lacrosse scandal. *Annals of Behavioral Medicine, 35*(1), 105–110.
33. Corrigan, P. (2004). How stigma interferes with mental health care. *The American Psychologist, 59*, 614–625. https://doi.org/10.1037/0003-066X.59.7.614
34. Pugh T, Hatzenbuehler M., Link B. Structural stigma and mental illness. Commissioned Paper for Committee on the Science of Changing Behavioral Health Social Norms, Mailman School of Public, Columbia University. Aug 2015.
35. Mental Illness. 2019. Retrieved 20 Oct 2020, from: https://www.nimh.nih.gov/health/statistics/mental-illness.shtml.
36. Schulze, B. (2007). Stigma and mental health professionals: A review of the evidence on an intricate relationship. *International Review of Psychiatry, 19*(2), 137–155.
37. Corrigan, P. W., Watson, A. C., Heyrman, M. L., Warpinski, A., Gracia, G., Slopen, N., & Hall, L. L. (2005). Structural stigma in state legislation. *Psychiatric Services, 56*(5), 557–563.
38. Bishop, T. F., Press, M. J., Keyhani, S., & Pincus, H. A. (2014). Acceptance of insurance by psychiatrists and the implications for access to mental health care. *JAMA Psychiatry, 71*(2), 176–181.
39. Cummings, J. R., Wen, H., Ko, M., & Druss, B. G. (2013). Geography and the Medicaid mental health care infrastructure: Implications for health care reform. *JAMA Psychiatry, 70*(10), 1084–1090.
40. McCleary-Gaddy, A. T., & Scales, R. (2019). Addressing mental illness stigma, implicit bias, and stereotypes in medical school. *Academic Psychiatry, 43*(5), 512–515.
41. Rada, R. E., & Johnson-Leong, C. (2004). Stress, burnout, anxiety and depression among dentists. *Journal of the American Dental Association (1939), 135*(6), 788–794.
42. Farrell, G. A. (2001). From tall poppies to squashed weeds: Why don't nurses pull together more? *Journal of Advanced Nursing, 35*, 26–33.
43. Arvaniti, A., Samakouri, M., Kalamara, E., Bochtsou, V., Bikos, C., & Livaditis, M. (2009). Health service staff's attitudes towards patients with mental illness. *Social Psychiatry and Psychiatric Epidemiology, 44*(8), 658–665.
44. Hampton, T. (2005). Experts address risk of physician suicide. *JAMA, 294*(10), 1189–1191.
45. Substance Abuse and Mental Health Services Administration. (2015). *Racial/ethnic Differences in mental health service use among adults. HHS publication no. SMA-15-4906.* Substance Abuse and Mental Health Services Administration. Retrieved from: http://www.integration.samhsa.gov/MHServicesUseAmongAdults.pdf
46. Alegria, M., Woo, M., Takeuchi, D., & Jackson, J. (2009). Ethnic and racial group-specific considerations. In P. Ruiz & A. Primm (Eds.), *Disparities in psychiatric care: Clinical and cross-cultural perspectives* (pp. 306–318). Lippincott Williams and Wilkins.
47. Paradies, Y., Ben, J., Denson, N., Elias, A., Priest, N., Pieterse, A., Gee, G., et al. (2015). Racism as a determinant of health: A systematic review and meta-analysis. *PLoS ONE, 10*, e0138511. https://doi.org/10.1371/journal.pone.0138511
48. Harrell, S. P. (2000). A multidimensional conceptualization of racism-related stress: Implications for the Well-being of people of color. *The American Journal of Orthopsychiatry, 70*(1), 42–57.
49. Williams, D. R., & Mohammed, S. A. (2013). Racism and health I: Pathways and scientific evidence. *The American Behavioral Scientist, 57*(8), 1152–1173.

50. Sawyer, P. J., Major, B., Casad, B. J., Townsend, S. S., & Mendes, W. B. (2012). Discrimination and the stress response: Psychological and physiological consequences of anticipating prejudice in interethnic interactions. *American Journal of Public Health, 102*(5), 1020–1026.
51. Korous, K. M., Causadias, J. M., & Casper, D. M. (2017). Racial discrimination and cortisol output: A meta-analysis. *Social Science & Medicine, 193*, 90–100.
52. Van Ryn, M., & Burke, J. (2000). The effect of patient race and socio-economic status on physicians' perceptions of patients. *Social Science & Medicine, 50*(6), 813–828.
53. Egede, L. E. (2006). Race, ethnicity, culture, and disparities in health care. *Journal of General Internal Medicine, 21*(6), 667.
54. Berz, J. P., Johnston, K., Backus, B., Doros, G., Rose, A. J., Pierre, S., & Battaglia, T. A. (2009). The influence of black race on treatment and mortality for early-stage breast cancer. *Medical Care, 47*(9), 986–992.
55. Cooper-Patrick, L., Gallo, J. J., Gonzales, J. J., Vu, H. T., Powe, N. R., Nelson, C., & Ford, D. E. (1999). Race, gender, and partnership in the patient-physician relationship. *JAMA, 282*(6), 583–589.
56. Silber, J. H., Rosenbaum, P. R., Romano, P. S., Rosen, A. K., Wang, Y., Teng, Y., Volpp, K. G., et al. (2009). Hospital teaching intensity, patient race, and surgical outcomes. *Archives of Surgery, 144*(2), 113–120.
57. Lee, C., Ayers, S. L., & Kronenfeld, J. J. (2009). The association between perceived provider discrimination, health care utilization, and health status in racial and ethnic minorities. *Ethnicity & Disease, 19*(3), 330.
58. Greer, T. M., Brondolo, E., & Brown, P. (2014). Systemic racism moderates effects of provider racial biases on adherence to hypertension treatment for African Americans. *Health Psychology, 33*(1), 35.
59. James. (2020b). Health and health-related correlates of internalized racism among racial/ethnic minorities: A review of the literature. *Journal of Racial and Ethnic Health Disparities, 7*(4), 785–806. https://doi.org/10.1007/s40615-020-00726-6
60. Hatter-Fisher, D., & Harper, W. (2017). The relevance of depression, alexithymia, and internalized racism to blood pressure in African Americans. *International Journal of Health and Social Sciences, 7*(1), 49–60.
61. James, D. (2020a). Self- and group-focused internalized racism, anxiety, and depression symptoms among African American adults: A core self-evaluation mediation pathway. *Group Processes & Intergroup Relations, 24*(8), 1335–1354. https://doi.org/10.1177/1368430220942849
62. Gale, M. M., Pieterse, A. L., Lee, D. L., Huynh, K., Powell, S., & Kirkinis, K. (2020). A meta-analysis of the relationship between internalized racial oppression and health-related outcomes. *The Counseling Psychologist, 48*(4), 498–525.
63. Gupta, A., Szymanski, D. M., & Leong, F. T. (2011). The "model minority myth": Internalized racialism of positive stereotypes as correlates of psychological distress, and attitudes toward help-seeking. *Asian American Journal of Psychology, 2*(2), 101–114.
64. Chae, D. H., Nuru-Jeter, A. M., Adler, N. E., Brody, G. H., Lin, J., Blackburn, E. H., & Epel, E. S. (2014). Discrimination, racial bias, and telomere length in African-American men. *American Journal of Preventive Medicine, 46*(2), 103–111.
65. McCabe, S. E., Hughes, T. L., Bostwick, W. B., West, B. T., & Boyd, C. J. (2009). Sexual orientation, substance use behaviors and substance dependence in the United States. *Addiction, 104*(8), 1333–1345. https://doi.org/10.1111/j.1360-0443.2009.02596.x
66. Lick, D. J., Durso, L. E., & Johnson, K. L. (2013). Minority stress and physical health among sexual minorities. *Perspectives on Psychological Science, 8*(5), 521–548. https://doi.org/10.1177/1745691613497965
67. King, M., Semlyen, J., Tai, S. S., Killaspy, H., Osborn, D., Popelyuk, D., & Nazareth, I. (2008). A systematic review of mental disorder, suicide, and deliberate self harm in lesbian, gay and bisexual people. *BMC Psychiatry, 8*, 70. https://doi.org/10.1186/1471-244X-8-70

68. Meyer, I. H. (2003). Prejudice, social stress, and mental health in lesbian, gay, and bisexual populations: Conceptual issues and research evidence. *Psychological Bulletin, 129*(5), 674–697. https://doi.org/10.1037/0033-2909.129.5.674
69. Mustanski, B., Andrews, R., & Puckett, J. A. (2016). The effects of cumulative victimization on mental health among lesbian, gay, bisexual, and transgender adolescents and young adults. *American Journal of Public Health, 106*(3), 527–533. https://doi.org/10.2105/AJPH.2015.302976
70. Evans-Polce, R. J., Veliz, P. T., Boyd, C. J., Hughes, T. L., & McCabe, S. E. (2020). Associations between sexual orientation discrimination and substance use disorders: Differences by age in US adults. *Social Psychiatry and Psychiatric Epidemiology, 55*(1), 101–110. https://doi.org/10.1007/s00127-019-01694-x
71. Yoshikawa, H., Alan-David Wilson, P., Chae, D. H., & Cheng, J. F. (2004). Do family and friendship networks protect against the influence of discrimination on mental health and HIV risk among Asian and Pacific islander gay men? *AIDS Education and Prevention, 16*(1), 84–100.
72. Li, C. C., Matthews, A. K., Aranda, F., Patel, C., & Patel, M. (2015). Predictors and consequences of negative patient-provider interactions among a sample of African American sexual minority women. *LGBT Health, 2*(2), 140–146.
73. Steele, L. S., Daley, A., Curling, D., Gibson, M. F., Green, D. C., Williams, C. C., & Ross, L. E. (2017). LGBT identity, untreated depression, and unmet need for mental health services by sexual minority women and trans-identified people. *Journal of Womens Health, 26*(2), 116–127.
74. Jabson, J. M., Mitchell, J. W., & Doty, S. B. (2016). Associations between non-discrimination and training policies and physicians' attitudes and knowledge about sexual and gender minority patients: A comparison of physicians from two hospitals. *BMC Public Health, 16*(1), 256.
75. Calabrese, S. K., Earnshaw, V. A., Krakower, D. S., Underhill, K., Vincent, W., Magnus, M., Dovidio, J. F., et al. (2018). A closer look at racism and heterosexism in medical students' clinical decision-making related to HIV pre-exposure prophylaxis (PrEP): Implications for PrEP education. *AIDS and Behavior, 22*(4), 1122–1138.
76. Turan, J. M., Elafros, M. A., Logie, C. H., Banik, S., Turan, B., Crockett, K. B., Murray, S. M., et al. (2019). Challenges and opportunities in examining and addressing intersectional stigma and health. *BMC Medicine, 17*(1), 7.
77. WHO Health Commission. (2008). *Final report of the CSDH*. World Health Organization.
78. Williams, D. R., Mohammed, S. A., Leavell, J., & Collins, C. (2010). Race, socioeconomic status and health: Complexities, ongoing challenges and research opportunities. *Annals of the New York Academy of Sciences, 1186*, 69.
79. Eisner, M. D., Blanc, P. D., Omachi, T. A., Yelin, E. H., Sidney, S., Katz, P. P., Iribarren, C., et al. (2011). Socioeconomic status, race and COPD health outcomes. *Journal of Epidemiology and Community Health, 65*(1), 26–34.
80. Stotzer, R. L. (2009). Violence against transgender people: A review of United States data. *Aggression and Violent Behavior, 14*(3), 170–179.
81. Williams, D. R., Lawrence, J. A., & Davis, B. A. (2019). Racism and health: Evidence and needed research. *Annual Review of Public Health, 40*, 105–125.
82. Mustillo, S., Krieger, N., Gunderson, E. P., Sidney, S., McCreath, H., & Kiefe, C. I. (2004). Self-reported experiences of racial discrimination and black–white differences in preterm and low-birthweight deliveries: The CARDIA study. *American Journal of Public Health, 94*(12), 2125–2131.
83. Tomfohr, L., Cooper, D. C., Mills, P. J., Nelesen, R. A., & Dimsdale, J. E. (2010). Everyday discrimination and nocturnal blood pressure dipping in black and white Americans. *Psychosomatic Medicine, 72*(3), 266.
84. Tesler, M. (2012). The spillover of racialization into health care: How President Obama polarized public opinion by racial attitudes and race. *American Journal of Political Science, 56*(3), 690–704.

85. Metzl, J. M. (2019). *Dying of whiteness: How the politics of racial resentment is killing America's heartland*. Hachette UK.
86. Siegel, J., Coleman, D. L., & James, T. (2018). Integrating social determinants of health into graduate medical education: A call for action. *Academic Medicine, 93*(2), 159–162.
87. Eisenberg, L., & Kleinman, A. (Eds.). (2012). *The relevance of social science for medicine* (Vol. 1). Springer Science & Business Media.
88. Himmelstein, M. S., Puhl, R. M., & Quinn, D. M. (2018). Weight stigma and health: The mediating role of coping responses. *Health Psychology, 37*(2), 139.

Asia T. McCleary-Gaddy, Ph.D. serves as the Director of Diversity and Inclusion for UTHealth and Assistant Professor of Psychiatry and Behavioral Sciences for McGovern Medical School. Asia serves the UTHealth community through design and implementation of policies and procedures that support diversity and inclusion, recruitment, and retention of URM faculty and students, program evaluation, and data analysis for students, residents, and faculty members. Dedicated to furthering the empirical research published on diversity and health, she has published in leading journals including Annals of Behavioral Medicine, Journal of Health Psychology, and Equality, Diversity, and Inclusion.

Previously, Dr. McCleary-Gaddy served as the inaugural Director of Diversity and Equity for Hackensack Meridian School of Medicine and helped launch the institution's high school pipeline/pathway programs. Prior to that role, she served as a Data Analyst for the Vermont Department of Health in Burlington, VT where she analyzed data for the Healthy People 2020 initiative. Dr. McCleary-Gaddy earned a PhD in Experimental Social Psychology. She also holds a Bachelor of Arts in Psychology with a distinction in Research and Creative Works from Rice University.

Drexler James, Ph.D. joined the faculty at Univeristy of Minnesota, Twin Cities in 2022. He completed his doctorate in Social Psychology from the University of Illinois at Chicago. Dr. James aims to advance theories of social stigma in ways that will help reduce persistent health disparities. Namely, rather than approaching stigmas as fixed "traits" that individuals possess, he examines stigma as a dynamic and relational social psychological process to reveal how it reinforces and reproduces health-relevant social inequality

Chapter 7
Transgender Health: The Present and the Future

Tukea L. Talbert

Transgender Healthcare: Can We Achieve High-Performing Healthcare Delivery to All?

"The performance of health systems in the United States falls far short of what is possible: It harms too often, costs too much, dissatisfies too many, and learns too slowly to perform well" ([1], p. 448). This statement is adapted from, "High Performance Health Care Delivery Systems: High Performance Toward What Purpose?" Dr. Peter Pronovost, a physician and industry leader in patient safety and quality of care, asserts that healthcare should help people thrive, prevent disease when feasible, commit to care when it cannot cure, and to cure when it cannot prevent.

Correspondingly, Ahluwalia et al. [2] outlined "dimensions of performance"—an evaluation framework used to identify high-performing healthcare delivery systems. The dimensions of performance include equity, access, patient experience, quality cost, and patient safety. Similarly, the Institute of Medicine's (IOM) Committee on Quality of Health Care in America identified six specific aims for healthcare improvement: safety, timely access, equity, effectiveness, patient-centeredness, and efficiency [3]. Although the "dimensions of performance" and IOM aims are each necessary for performance improvement of healthcare systems, they do not account for dimensions of healthcare that disproportionately affect populations such as transgender individuals (TI) who experience structural stigma, discrimination, and marginalization when seeking healthcare.

T. L. Talbert (✉)
Office of Executive VP for Health Affairs, University of Kentucky HealthCare,
Lexington, KY, USA
e-mail: Tukea.talbert@uky.edu

© The Author(s), under exclusive license to Springer Nature
Switzerland AG 2023
R. Scales, A. T. McCleary-Gaddy (eds.), *Cultural Issues in Healthcare*,
https://doi.org/10.1007/978-3-031-20826-3_7

Research also asserts that there may be additional factors, guided by healthcare professionals that drive the "dimensions of performance." These include care coordination, community service, innovation, and organizational responsiveness [2]. To achieve key dimensions of quality care, and especially the (IOM) goals of equity and access, healthcare professionals must care for the diverse patient population, which includes the transgender population.

This chapter will focus on (1) transgender healthcare research and challenges, (2) unique healthcare issues experienced by the transgender population, (3) structural stigma and discrimination experienced by transgender individuals, and (4) the next steps to address gaps in research, education, and clinical practice to improve overall access to care by transgender individuals. This chapter will highlight how healthcare systems and members of the healthcare team (inclusive of providers, nurses, clinicians, administrators, and leadership) may unconsciously and consciously eliminate possibilities of progress in care delivery for TIs. Notably, this chapter promulgates thinking outside the proverbial box and identifying how to become more intentionally responsive and innovative when caring for transgender patients.

Background

Transgender is a "catch-all" term used to define individuals whose gender expression or identity varies from the culturally bound gender associated with one's natal sex or birth sex (i.e., male or female) [4, 5]. Several terms are used by TIs to define their gender identity such as woman, man, genderqueer, transgender man, transgender woman, bi-gender, and butch queen [5]. Transgender individuals have multiple ways that they choose to socially transition their gender identity and/or expression that includes changing their name, pronoun(s), and/or undergoing medical transition interventions that include surgery (gender-affirming surgery) and/or cross-sex hormones [4]. Other individuals may decide to have a gender identity or expression outside of the conventional gender binary (male vs. female) and are considered gender non-binary people [4].

Because of the variability of transgender categorization, many different projections exist to quantify the population size. One source projects that 0.03–0.05% of the US population is transgender [6–8]. Other sources such as the UCLA School of Law state that within the United States, an estimated 0.3% of adults identify as transgender [7]. This implies that the number of transgender people may be different depending on how the data are retrieved through self-identification or projections. Herman et al. [9] state that recent studies predict that 0.7% of US youth between the ages of 13–17-years old identify as transgender and 3.2% of US high school students are uncertain of their gender identity [10]. Winter and researchers (2016) speculate that approximately 25 million transgender people exist worldwide with approximately 1.4 million in the US who identify as transgender. Notably, these numbers vary due to the overarching umbrella of transgender as a term and inconsistencies in the inclusion of transgender in various census surveillance tools and processes. Recent literature suggests that researchers frequently use convenience samples or subgroups who seek gender-affirming care as a means to project the population size [11]. It is noteworthy to say that numbers from subgroups drastically underestimate the size of the larger population of TIs who are unable or choose not to access this specialty care [11].

The issues with TIs' healthcare, healthcare access, and the achievement of optimal outcomes are multifactorial. Factors that contribute to many of these issues include the dearth of research available on the transgender population's health, structural stigma, social stereotyping and discrimination within the healthcare system, and a lack of formal training and programs (education and work environment) for members of the healthcare team—most notably physicians and nurses.

Research

In a literature review conducted over two decades (1980–1999), Boehmer [12] found that only 0.1% of all indexed articles in MEDLINE focused on LGBT health. More than half (56%) of that volume focused on HIV and STDs among primarily gay and bisexual men. Historically, a large focus of LGBT research has been among white bisexual and gay men. Little is known about other non-white bisexual and gay individuals and even less about the transgender population and the intersection of people of color (POC) [13]. Edminston et al. [14] conducted a systemic review of the literature published between 2001 and 2015 to investigate the number and breadth of articles that focused on preventative health services for TIs. The review identified 1304 eligible studies. However, only 41 discussed transgender primary or preventative care. Out of the 41 articles focusing on the transgender population, the majority of studies focused on HIV rates and risk behaviors, with a few articles also addressing pelvic examinations, insurance coverage, tobacco use, and cholesterol screening [12]. No studies addressed routine preventive screenings such as colorectal screenings, flu shots, mammography, or chest/breast examinations. This gap in research on primary care and prevention for TIs may put them at risk for certain cancers if their natal sex organs are not routinely screened.

To date, one of the strongest and most thorough reviews of existing literature on transgender population health is the work conducted by Reisner et al. [15]. Researchers reviewed and synthesized peer-reviewed literature performed over an 8-year (2008–2014) period. Their inclusion criteria consisted of three elements: (1) studies published between January 1, 2008 and December 20, 2014; (2) studies published in English, French, or Spanish; and (3) any study design inclusive of quantitative data related to disease burden in transgender individuals of all ages.

Their review identified 116 studies over 30 countries with most of the research available in the United States. The most commonly used study design was cross-sectional (78% of studies) with slightly under 3% being interventional studies. Most of the studies used convenience sampling methods as opposed to randomization. The following six health outcome domains were developed from 981 unique health-related data points: (1) mental health, (2) sexual and reproductive health, (3) substance use, (4) violence and victimization, (5) stigma and discrimination, and (6) general health outcomes. The health outcomes were listed in order of the frequency cited among the 981 unique health-related data points [16].

Mental health represented the most commonly studied area of the transgender population (N = 303 data points, 31%) with the majority of the focus on mood disorders (32%) [15]. Some of the specific challenges and study limitations include inconsistent operationalization of depression. The analysis showed a need for additional research on posttraumatic stress disorders since it is well-known that many transgender individuals experience victimization and violence [15].

Sexual and reproductive health is the second most studied domain (N = 219 data points, 22%). Of the 219 data points, human immunodeficiency virus (HIV) or sexually transmitted infections (STIs) prevalence represents 75% (163 of 219) of the sexual and reproductive health outcomes. Reisner et al. [15] noted that the focus on STIs and HIV demonstrates a focus on TIs assigned male sex at birth. As noted earlier, approximately 0.3% of adults (90,000 individuals) are transgender in the United States [11]. TIs have many complex healthcare needs that range from high rates of sexual, mental, and physical risks that are complicated further by poor access to healthcare services [17]. As previously discussed, the sexual health issues that have received the most attention from researchers include the prevalence of HIV, acquired immunodeficiency syndrome (AIDS), and other sexually transmitted infections [18–20]. Factors associated with high HIV/AIDS rates with TIs include sex work, multiple partners, early sexual experiences, needle sharing to administer cross-sex hormones, and random sexual encounters [16, 21]. The risk of HIV/AIDS is especially high for transgender females and those of African American race [16, 21].

Future research should aim to investigate the impact of making hormone therapy more available to TIs and its effect on the prevalence and incidence of HIV. This review also suggests that other sexual and reproductive health concerns receive little to no attention in research on transgender populations. To promote holistic healthcare, more research is needed on reproductive health, options for storing eggs/sperm, and prevention of STIs/HIV.

Another shortfall exists in the paucity of information about health issues affecting LGBT populations in Healthy People 2010 (HP, 2010). Although Healthy People 2010 included health objectives directed towards sexual orientation, data were not collected to track those objectives [13]. The document not only failed to identify specific health objectives to eliminate health disparities among the LGBT population, but it entirely overlooked gender identity and expression and the transgender population [22]. This clearly indicates a design deficit within the Healthy People 2010, platform. While the intention was promising, the omission of a plan of measurement along with the lack of inclusion of identity and expression will result in no data to support progress with TIs.

After sexual and reproductive health, substance use was the third most commonly studied domain for TIs (N = 193 data points, 20%). The most frequently studied subsets include alcohol, marijuana, tobacco, and illicit drug use. On the contrary, very little attention was focused on substance abuse and dependence (N = 10 data points, 1%) [15].

Like sexual orientation, gender identity and gender expression traverse all race/ethnic and socioeconomic groups. Because of the small size and large diversity within the transgender population, representative sampling in research is difficult [13]. In summary, research drives practice, optimal outcomes, and generates new knowledge. Very little transgender health research exists; and within what does exist, access to general healthcare is among the least researched fields [23]. Research trends show that many opportunities exist in regard to the amount and areas of focus for studies about the transgender population. However, it is pivotal that future research addresses the standardization of how transgender individuals are identified, inconsistencies with operationalizing transgender in terms of what falls under the transgender umbrella methodology issues predominantly regarding sampling techniques, and the use of a cross-sectional study design with few interventional studies (<3%) [15].

Structural Stigma

A growing body of literature supports discrimination and stigma as a basic source of health disparities [24–27], which is a cornerstone of health inequity. TIs are frequently socially marginalized as a result of rejection by families and communities due to their gender expression and/or gender identity [28]. Structural stigma refers to institutional practices and laws, environmental conditions, and societal norms that restrict resources, opportunities, and the welfare of stigmatized individuals [29]. Power, which is arguably the nucleus of structural stigma, is used by the majority to marginalize those who are different [30]. Under a binary system, having a gender identity or expression concordant with one's sex characteristics is viewed as socially normative, while transgender individuals are classified as "other" [31, 32]. The societal view that the population can only be placed in two gender categories based on one's natal sex perpetuates the structural stigma that TIs are non-normative and the cisgender majority is considered the "normal gender" of privilege and power.

Transgender population health and access are affected by the structural stigma within a society through practices and policies that limit healthcare access. TIs are not currently covered under most insurance mechanisms, which may be related to the higher prevalence of unemployment, which itself is likely due to employment discrimination [6, 33]. Khan [34] highlights that even when insured, TIs face barriers to accessing gender-affirming care. Private insurers often refer to gender-affirming medical interventions as preexisting, medically unnecessary, or cosmetic as grounds to exclude coverage [34]. This may result in many individuals paying out of pocket for care, which in some cases is cost-prohibitive [34].

Another form of structural stigma that impacts TIs' access to healthcare is the lack of insurance coverage and/or the perception of inadequate coverage. Lack of coverage may be directly linked in part to joblessness and poverty, which is prevalent among TIs [30, 35].

It is noteworthy to state that structural stigma creates an environment that promotes minoritization at the interpersonal and individual levels, which may be even more stigmatizing to patients. This is relevant because the latter involves frontline staffers, often in healthcare, at the point of service that interacts with TIs. These are leaders and healthcare workers who operate with their personal biases, which may be promulgated by policies and other structural limitations within the practice settings. Sitkin and Murota [36] affirm that a rigid binary exists within the US and those whose sex assigned at birth is believed discordant with their gender identity or expression face significant stigma.

Stigma and discrimination are the fifth most frequently studied domain among transgender individuals (N = 93 data points, 9.5%). This area is of significance because it relates directly to the healthcare environment and its impact on access, patient–provider relationships (provider inclusive or MDs, RNs, other clinicians), and the overall quality of healthcare [15]. Slightly over half of the studies (54%) specifically address stigma and discrimination in the healthcare milieu [15]. Discrimination and stigma are evidenced in ways ranging from care denial to postponement of care. Reisner et al. [15] point out that despite these findings, there is a paucity of literature on the impact of interventions designed to decrease stigma and discrimination against the transgender population.

Recent studies continue to demonstrate structural stigma that exists in healthcare against TIs. In addition to structural, interpersonal, and individual stigma, data show that a lack of preparation, training, and education of nurses and physicians to care for TIs create barriers to care. Surprisingly, nursing has been slower than other health professionals to address LGBT health [37]. Only a small number of studies have researched the attitudes of nursing students, nurse educators, and nurses [38, 39]. Despite the research, nurses frequently state they are comfortable caring for LGBT patients; and express no need for training because they "treat everyone the same" [40].

Johnston and Shearer [41] found that few data exist in the specialty of internal medicine graduate medical education (GME) regarding the provision of comprehensive care to transgender individuals. While this study focused on internal medicine GME, other studies support this lack of training and preparation in medical schools across the United States and Canada. The primary focus of any education provided, which averages 5 h or less is about teaching students to ask about the gender of patients' sexual partners [42]. Reisner et al. [15] conclude that there needs to be more research conducted on stigma and discrimination in order to improve healthcare access to TIs.

Unique Healthcare Needs

High rates of depression, substance abuse, self-harm, and suicide among TIs are well documented in the literature [17, 35, 43–45]. The risk of suicide is perceived to be worse among children and youth with gender dysphoria (GD), which is defined as a marked incongruence between their assigned gender (related to natal sex) and their expressed gender [46]. Data on completed suicides among youth with GD are unknown; however, clinicians assert that they are critically high [47]. To complicate matters more, LGBT individuals have a documented high risk of familial maltreatment as compared to heterosexual persons [48].

Familial behaviors, treatment, and attitudes have been linked to the mental health and well-being of transgender youth [48]. It is estimated that 575,000 to 1.6 million US youth live without a home and without a family [49]. One study estimates that between 30% and 40% of homeless youth identify as TIs, lesbian, gay, or bisexual [50]. Transgender youths are more likely to be homeless and more than twice as likely to attempt suicide [51]. Homeless transgender adolescents experience more sexual victimization, physical and mental health issues ranging from suicidality, posttraumatic stress disorder, and depression [42]. Reisner et al. [15] also found that transgender youth experience a high prevalence of mental health disorders, which include major depressive disorders (35.4%) and suicidality (20.2%) [15]. The mental health issues among transgender youth place them at risk for other challenges such as substance use. The prevalence of substance use is two and a half to four times greater for transgender adolescents compared with their non-transgender counterparts [52].

Next Steps: How to Create a High-Performing Healthcare Delivery System for Transgender Patients

Over the last decade, the transgender population has grown [30]. While growth typically makes an entity more visible, transgender individuals have fallen victim to the "Erasure Concept"; hence, becoming less visible in some ways. Erasure is "a defining condition of how transgender is managed in culture and institutions, a condition that ultimately inscribes transgender as impossible" ([53], pp. 4–5). This concept exists because transgender individuals are denied an appropriate legal identity concordant with their gender identity and expression [54]. The concept of erasure is perpetuated through numerous structural forms of stigma that exist globally, nationally, and locally. It is most prominent in healthcare where TIs experience a lack of insurance and/or adequate coverage for transgender-specific care/gender-affirming care, hostility, and clinicians who lack training and education on transgender-specific care.

Reisner et al. [15] highlighted the impact of "gendered situated vulnerabilities." These vulnerabilities are related to the ways in which health is shaped by the distribution of power associated with gender [55, 56]. The way forward must include a deeper understanding of the role and impact of sexed and gendered contexts and how they place TIs at risk [26, 57]. Several organizations including the World Professional Association for Transgender Health (WPATH) recommend a two-step method with data collection as a means to better understand sexed and gendered contexts and their associated power alignment and their influence on risks affiliated with transgender individuals' health inequities. The process looks at natal sex (male vs. female) and gender identity (man, woman, transgender, genderqueer, etc.). Overall, in the research arena, policymakers and healthcare leaders will need qualitative, quantitative, and many more interventional studies with sound experimental designs to create policies and develop best practices respectively to meet the needs of the transgender population.

Power, privilege, and access are key variables impacted by structural racism, social determinants of health (SDoH) , and long-term minoritization of transgender patients. The path forward must be focused on the dismantling of structural racism and associated stigma with TIs. This will require intentional efforts to adequately prepare healthcare workers who can provide culturally sensitive care, which has to start with medical education curriculums structured to equip doctors, nurses, and other healthcare workers to take care of transgender patients. Healthcare facilities have to be committed to furthering training on the provision of patient-centered care of TIs that includes all disciplines and reinforced on a routine basis to include proper use of pronouns; the use of preferred names by patients; and gender-neutral language [58]. The latter is really only touching the surface of what it means to create equal access to quality health for transgender patients.

This chapter has focused on research opportunities, structural stigma, and barriers that TIs encounter with healthcare access. Insurance challenges, healthcare workers' lack of transgender care competency and personal prejudices, and a post-secondary education system that is not centered on preparing healthcare professionals to provide culturally sensitive care to all people all contribute to the issues plaguing the TI community. Healthcare systems must create transgender-affirming policies and structures that have zero tolerance for bigotry, prejudice, and discrimination based on an individual's gender identity and gender expression.

When transgender patients have safe psychological spaces to express their true feelings, concerns, and challenges, care can be targeted to meet specific needs in a way that patients will not only be treated but also seen, heard, and understood [58]. Systems need to be redesigned so that TIs can have a place that has LGBTQ friendly healthcare workers and provide more comprehensive multidisciplinary care that includes primary care, surgical consultations (gynecology, plastics, urology), cancer screenings, and psychiatric services to address the multifaceted nature of their needs [14].

Healthcare providers and leaders must find innovative ways to engage transgender patients in their care and future direction. In a study conducted by Poteat et al. [59], they found that interpersonal stigma (everyday interactions with others) functions to reinforce the medical hierarchy and power when providers face uncertainty. This study also suggests that uncertainty and ambivalence displayed by physicians during patient encounters are transparent to transgender patients. These factors inhibit the ability to build a therapeutic, trusting relationship between patients and their providers.

Healthy People 2020 defines health equity as the "attainment of the highest level of health for all people." This requires valuing everyone equally and addressing avoidable inequalities between populations. This is the goal for healthcare generally, and all those individuals in positions of leadership, authority, and power to impact the future of healthcare as they work to eliminate avoidable, remedial, and unjust health inequalities. Healthcare organizations must hold each other accountable to adopt best practices for transgender-specific care and to create policies that have zero tolerance for hostility and/or discrimination against individuals who belong to sexual or gender minorities [41]. The healthcare team must embrace industry standards that have been developed by experts and innovators regarding transgender care (see Table 7.1). Healthcare teams have the power to define what a high-performing healthcare delivery system looks like, and it has to include the creation of care systems and models of care that ensure the highest level of health for all people.

Table 7.1 Transgender healthcare resources

Resource	Description	Source[a]
University of Louisville LGBT health certificate program	Interdisciplinary approach to increase LGBT training for students in the School of Medicine, nursing, dentistry, public health, and information sciences; it is offered as an extracurricular course over lunch break with a total offering of 11 sessions	www.educationforhealth.net [60]
Association of American Medical Colleges (AAMC)	In 2014, the AAMC released a report intended to assist medical schools with the integration of elements regarding transgender cultural competency at the curricular and institutional levels	http://bit.ly/1DKyzBj [61], pp. 1786
World Professional Association for Transgender Health (WPATH)	This is an interdisciplinary (nonprofit) professional and educational organization devoted to transgender health. *Mission:* To promote evidenced-based care, education, research, advocacy, public policy, and respect for transgender health. *Vision:* To bring together diverse professionals dedicated to developing best practices and supportive policies worldwide that promote health, research, education, respect, dignity, and equality for transgender, trans-sexual, and gender-variant people in all cultural settings	www.wpath.org
Centerlink-the community of LGBT Centers	"Centerlink is a member-based coalition of LGBT community centers with the goals of helping improve their organizational and service delivery capacities, increasing awareness of national issues and access to public resources, and advancing the rights of LGBT individuals"	http://www.lgbtcenters.org [62], p. 397

Center of excellence for transgender health	"It is housed at the University of California, san Francisco, and develops programs to improve the overall health and well-being of transgenderindividuals"	http://www.transhealth.ucsf.edu/trans?page=home-00-00 [62], p. 397
Centers for Disease Control and Prevention (CDC)-lesbian, gay, bisexual, and transgender health	"The site provides extensive, excellent quality information about LGBT issues aimed at laypersons, healthcare providers, public health professionals, and students"	http://www.cdc.gov/lgbthealth/index.htm [62], p. 397
Gay and Lesbian Medical Association (GLMA)	"It is a nonprofit member organization of LGBT healthcare professionals with the mission of ensuring equality in healthcare for LGBT patients and professionals and providing related public policy advocacy"	http://glma.org/ [62], p. 397
Healthcare equality index-creating a National Standard for equal treatment of LGBT patients and their families	"It is a voluntary annual survey of healthcare policies and practices related to LGBT patients and their families. It is performed by the human rights campaign"	www.hrc.org/hei [62], p. 398
Healthy People 2020	"This is an initiative of multiple US government agencies which establish ambitions yet achievable 10-year objectives for improving the nation's health. They have 42 objectives, including a new one of improving health, safety, and well-being of LGBT individuals"	http://www.healthypeople.gov/2020/topicsobjectives2020/overview.aspx?topicid=25 [62], p. 398
MedlinePlus	"It is the National Library of Medicine's consumer health site. It is a site that collects high-quality patient-level health information and includes hundreds of health topics pages with recommended websites including LGBT health issues"	http://www.nlm.nih.gov/medlineplus/gaylesbianandtranasgenderhealthth.html [62], p. 399

(continued)

Table 7.1 (continued)

Resource	Description	Source[a]
National coalition for LGBT health	"It is a federal level advocacy establishment made up of member organizations dedicated to increasing knowledge about LGBT populations' health status, improving their access to healthcare services, enhancing professional and cultural competency in those providing healthcare services to LGBT individuals."	http://lgbthealth.weboutionary.com/ [62], p 0.399
The joint commission (TJC) seven healthcare Centers (location): Lyon Martin health services (San Francisco, CA), LA LGBT Center (Los Angeles, CA), Howard Brown health Center (Chicago, IL), Mazzoni Center (Philadelphia, PA), Whitman Walker health (Washington, DC), Callen Lorde community health Center (New York, NY), Fenway health (Boston, MA)	TJC developed a roadmap for hospitals to improve effective communication, cultural competence, and patient/family-centered care in 2020. Based on expert opinion and comprehensive research, investigators consider these centers to be providers of comprehensive healthcare to LGBT individuals, participants in LGBT advocacy, and providers of education for LGBT health	http://www.jointcommission.org/assets/1/6/ARoadmapforHospitalsfinalversion727.pdf [63]

Note. In Table 7.1 I provide specific transgender healthcareresources that have been compiled by field experts in transgender healthcare. The resources range from academic certificate programs, various helpful links and websites, to healthcare centers that are known for providing comprehensive transgender healthcare. Healthcare teams do not need to "reinvent the wheel" but they would be remiss to not use these resources to "roll" forward. Every patient deserves the right to autonomy and self-determination [64] and the healthcare team is well-positioned to facilitate and safeguard that right. The time to act is now and healthcare teams must do what is just and within the scope of providing safe and quality care at the highest level of health for all people. As opposed to being the barrier to care for transgender individuals, healthcare teams should be the key to access healthcare that is gender-specific and appropriate to meet their unique needs. Healthcare needs to use the momentum created by the recent decision made by the US Supreme Court regarding the protection of LGBTQ individuals under Title VII of the 1964 Civil Rights Act. The newly appointed US Justice, Neil Gorsuch, stated "The law's ban on job discrimination on the basis of 'sex' means that firing employees or not hiring them because of their sexual orientation or gender identity is illegal (latimes.com, accessed online 7/26/2020)." This was a bold action taken on June 15, 2020, to expand this protection to LGBTQ Americans. Just as in the workplace, the healthcare system must ensure that all patients are given a fair opportunity to achieve their highest health potential

[a] Full sources listed in reference section

References

1. Pronovost, P. (2017). High-performing healthcare delivery systems: High performance toward what purpose? *Joint Commission Journal on Quality and Patient Safety, 43*(9), 448–449. https://doi.org/10.1016/j.jcjq.2017.06.001
2. Ahluwalia, S., Damberg, C. A., Silverman, M., Motala, A., & Shekelle, P. (2017). What defines a high-performing health care delivery system: A systematic review. *Joint Commission Journal on Quality and Patient Safety, 43*(9), 450–459. https://doi.org/10.1016/j.jcjq.2017.03.010
3. Institute of Medicine [IOM]. (2001). *Crossing the quality chasm: A new health system for the 21st century.* National Academies Press.
4. Davidson, M. (2007). Seeking refuge under the umbrella: Inclusion, exclusion, and organizing within the category transgender. *Sexuality Research & Social Policy, 4*(4), 60–80. https://doi.org/10.1525/srsp.2007.4.4.60
5. Valentine, D. (2007). *Imagining transgender: An ethnography of a category.* Duke University Press.
6. Conron, K. J., Scott, G., Stowell, G. S., & Landers, S. J. (2012). Transgender health in Massachusetts: Results from a household probability sample of adults. *American Journal of Public Health, 102*(1), 118–122. https://doi.org/10.2105/AJPH.2011.300315
7. Gates, G. J. (2011). *How many people are lesbian, gay, bisexual and transgender?* The Williams Institute, UCLA School of Law. https://www.ciis.edu//Documents/PDFs/PublicPrograms/ExpandingtheCircle/How-many-people-are- LGBT-Final.pdf
8. Reisner, S. L., Conron, K. J., Tardiff, L. A., Jarvis, S., Gordon, A. R., & Austin, S. B. (2014). Monitoring the health of transgender and gender minority populations: Validity of natal sex and gender identity survey items in all national cohorts of young adults. *BMC Public Health, 14*(1), 1224–1234.
9. Herman, J. L., Flores, A. R., Brown, T. N. T., Wilson, B. D. M., & Conron, K. J. (2017). *Age of individuals who identify as transgender in the United States.* The Williams Institute, UCLA School of Law. Retrieved from: https://williamsinstitute.law.ucla.edu/wpcontent/uploads/TransAgeReport.pdf.
10. Kann, L., Olsen, E. D., McManus, T., Harris, W. A., Shanklin, S. L., Flint, K. H., Zaza, S., et al. (2016). Sexual identity, sex of sexual contacts, and health-related behaviors among students in grades 9-12 - United States and selected sites, 2015. *Morbidity and Mortality Weekly Report. Surveillance Summaries, 65*(9), 1–202. https://doi.org/10.15585/mmwr.ss6509a1
11. Winter, S., Diamond, M., Green, J., Karasic, D., Reed, T., Whittle, S., & Wylie, K. (2016). Transgender people: Health at the margins of society. *Lancet, 388*(10042), 390–400. https://doi.org/10.1016/S0140-6736(16)00683-8
12. Boehmer, U. (2002). Twenty years of public health research: Inclusion of lesbian, gay, bisexual, and transgender populations. *American Journal of Public Health, 92*(7), 1125–1130. https://doi.org/10.2105/AJPH.92.7.1125
13. Harcourt, J. (2006). Current issues in lesbian, gay, bisexual, and transgender (LGBT) health. *Journal of Homosexuality, 51*(1), 1–11. https://doi.org/10.1300/J082v51n01_01
14. Edminston, E. K., Donald, C. A., Sattler, A. R., Peebles, J. K., Ehrenfeld, J. M., & Eckstrand, K. L. (2016). Opportunities and gaps in primary care preventative health services for transgender patients: A systemic review. *Transgender Health, 1*(1), 216–230. https://doi.org/10.1089/trgh.2016.0019
15. Reisner, S. L., Biello, K. B., White Hughto, J. M., Kuhns, L., Mayer, K. H., Garofalo, R., & Mimiaga, M. J. (2016). Psychiatric diagnoses and comorbidities in a diverse, multicity cohort of young transgender women: Baseline findings from project life skills. *Journal of American Medical Association Pediatrics, 170*(5), 481–486. https://doi.org/10.1001/jamapediatrics.2016.0067
16. Reisner, S. L., Perkovich, B., & Mimiago, M. J. (2010). A mixed methods study of the sexual health needs of New England transmen who have sex with nontransgender men. *AIDS Patient Care and STDs, 24*(8), 1–14. https://doi.org/10.1089/apc.2010.0059

17. Institute of Medicine [IOM]. (2011). *The health of lesbian, gay, bisexual, and transgender people: Building a foundation for better understanding*. The National Academies Press. http://www.nap.edu/catalog.php?record_id=13128

18. Giani, A., & LeBail, J. (2011). HIV infection and STI in the transpopulation: A critical review. *Revue D'Epidemiologie Et De Sante Publique, 59*(4), 259–268. https://doi.org/10.1016/j.respe.2011.02.102

19. Grant, J. M., Mottet, L. A., Tanis, J., Harrison, J., Herman, J. L., & Keisling, M. (2010). *National transgender discrimination survey report on health and health care*. US Transgender Survey.

20. Herbst, J. H., Jacobs, E. D., Finlayson, T. S., McKleroy, V. S., Newmann, S. P., & Crepaz, N. (2007). Estimating HIV prevalence and risk behaviors of transgender persons in the United States: A systemic review. *Journal of AIDS Behavior, 2*(1), 1–17. https://doi.org/10.1007/s10461-007-9299-3

21. Lindley, L. L., Nicholson, T. J., Kerby, M. B., & Lu, N. (2003). HIV/STI associated risk behaviors among self-identified lesbian, gay, bisexual, and transgender college students in the United States. *AIDS Education and Prevention, 15*(5), 413–429. https://doi.org/10.1521/aeap.15.6.413.24039

22. Sell, R. L., & Baker, J. B. (2001). Sexual orientation data collection and progress toward healthy people 2010. *American Journal of Public Health, 91*(6), 876–882. https://doi.org/10.2105/AJPH.91.6.876

23. Lo, S., & Horton, R. (2016). Transgender health: An opportunity for global health equity. *Lancet, 388*(10042), 316–318. https://doi.org/10.1016/S0140-6736(16)30675-4

24. Krieger, N. (1999). Embodying inequality: A review of concepts, measure, and methods for studying health consequences of discrimination. *International Journal of Health Services, 29*(2), 295–352. https://doi.org/10.2190/M11W-VWXE-KQM9-G97Q

25. Krieger, N. (2012). Methods for the scientific study of discrimination and health: An ecosocial approach. *American Journal of Public Health, 102*(5), 936–944. https://doi.org/10.2105/AJPH.2011.300544

26. Link, B. G., & Phelan, J. C. (1995). Social conditions as fundamental causes of disease. *Journal of Health and Social Behavior, 35*, 80–94. https://doi.org/10.2307/2626958

27. Meyer, I. H., & Northridge, M. E. (2007). Prejudice and discrimination as social stressors. In I. H. Meyer & M. E. Northridge (Eds.), *The health of sexual minorities: Public health perspectives on lesbian, gay, bisexual, and transgender populations* (pp. 242–267). Springer Science + Business Media.

28. Rodriquez, A., Agardh, A., & Asamoah, B. O. (2018). Self-reported discrimination in health-care settings based on recognizability as transgender: A cross-sectional study among transgender U.S. citizens. *Archives of Sexual Behavior, 47*(4), 973–985. https://doi.org/10.1007/s10508017-1028-z

29. Hatzenbuehler, M. L., McLaughlin, K. A., Keyes, K. M., & Hasin, D. S. (2010). The impact of institutional discrimination on psychiatric disorders in lesbian, gay and bisexual populations: A prospective study. *American Journal of Public Health, 100*(3), 452–459. https://doi.org/10.2105/AJPH.2009.168815

30. White Hughto, J. M., Reisner, S. L., & Pachankis, J. E. (2015). Transgender stigma and health: A critical review of stigma determinants, mechanisms, and interventions. *Social Science & Medicine, 147*, 222–231. https://doi.org/10.1016/j.socscimed.2015.11.010

31. Link, B. G., & Phelan, J. C. (2014). Stigma power. *Social Science & Medicine, 103*, 24–32. https://doi.org/10.1016/j.socscimed.2013.07.035

32. Schilt, K., & Westbrook, L. (2009). Doing gender, doing heteronormativity: Gender normal, transgender people, and the social maintenance of heterosexuality. *Gender and Society, 23*(4), 440–464. https://doi.org/10.1177/0891243209340034

33. Grant, J. M., Mottet, L. A., Tanis, J., Harrison, J., Herman, J. L., & Keisling, M. (2011). *Injustice at every turn: A report of the national transgender discrimination survey*. National Center for Transgender Equality and National Gay and Lesbian Task Force.

34. Khan, L. (2013). Transgender health at the crossroads: Legal norms, insurance markets, and the threat of healthcare reform. *Yale Journal of Health Policy, Law, and Ethics, 11*(2), 375–418.
35. Xavier, J. M., Hannold, J. A., Bradford, J., & Simmons, R. (2007). *The health, health-related needs, and life course experiences of transgender Virginians*. Virginia Department of Health. https://doi.org/10.1037/e544442014-001
36. Sitkin, N., & Murota, D. (2017). Moving beyond the basics of the binary: Addressing mental health needs and suicidality among transgender youth. *Journal of the American Academy of Child and Adolescent Psychiatry, 56*(9), 725–726. https://doi.org/10.1016/j.jaac.2017.07.005
37. Eliason, M. J., DeJoseph, J., & Dibble, S. D. (2010). Nursing's' silence about lesbian, gay, bisexual, and transgender issues: The need for emancipatory efforts. *Advances in Nursing Science, 33*(3), 206–218. https://doi.org/10.1097/ANS.0b013e3181e63e49
38. Blackwell, C. (2007). Belief in the "free choice" model of homosexuality: A correlate of homophobia in registered nurses. *Journal of LGBT Health Research, 3*(3), 31–40. https://doi.org/10.1080/15574090802093117
39. Dinkel, S., Patzel, B., McGuire, M. J., Rolfe, E., & Purcell, K. (2007). Measures of homophobia among nursing students and faculty: A midwestern perspective. *International Journal of Journal of Nursing Scholarship, 4*, 24. https://doi.org/10.2202/1548-923X.1491
40. Beagan, B. L., Frederick, E., & Goldberg, L. (2012). Nurses' work with LGBTQ patients: "They're just like everybody else, so what's the difference?". *The Canadian Journal of Nursing Research, 44*(3), 44–63.
41. Johnston, C. D., & Shearer, L. S. (2017). Internal medicine resident attitudes, prior education, comfort, and knowledge regarding delivering comprehensive primary care to transgender patients. *Transgender Health, 2*(1), 91–95. https://doi.org/10.1089/trgh.2017.0007
42. McBride, D. (2012). Homelessness and health care disparities among lesbian, gay, bisexual, and transgender youth. *Journal of Pediatric Nursing, 27*(2), 177–179. https://doi.org/10.1016/j.pedn.2011.11.007
43. Burgess, D., Lee, R., Tran, A., & Ryn, M. (2007). Effects of perceived discrimination on mental health and mental health services utilization among gay, lesbian, bisexual, and transgender persons. *Journal of LGBT Health Research, 3*(4), 1–15. https://doi.org/10.1080/15574090802226626
44. Duhon, L., Koenig, K., & Fennie, K. (2008). Gynecologic care of the female-to-male transgender man. *Journal of Midwifery & Women's Health, 53*(4), 331–337. https://doi.org/10.1016/j.jmwh.2008.02.003
45. Scourfield, J., Roen, K., & McDermott, L. (2008). Lesbian, gay, bisexual, and transgender young people's experiences of distress: Resilience, ambivalence, and self-destructive behavior. *Health & Social Care in the Community, 16*(3), 329–336.
46. American Psychiatric Association [APA]. (2013). *Diagnostic and statistical manual of mental disorders* (5th ed.). American Psychiatric Publishing. https://doi.org/10.1176/appi.books.9780890425596
47. Karasic, D., & Ehrensaft, D. (2015). *We must put an end to gender conversion therapy for kids*. WIRED. http://www.wired.com/2015/07/must-put-end-gender-convesion-therapy kids/
48. Ryan, C., Huebner, P., Diaz, R. M., & Sanchez, J. (2009). Family rejection as a predictor of negative health outcomes in White and Latino lesbian, gay, and bisexual young adults. *Pediatrics, 123*, 346–352. https://doi.org/10.1542/peds.2007-3524
49. National Center on Family Homelessness. State report card on childhood homelessness: America's youngest outcasts. 2009. http://www.homelesschildrenamerica.org/findings.php.
50. Corliss, H. L., Goodenow, C. S., Nichols, L., & Austin, S. B. (2011). High burden of homelessness among sexual minority adolescents: Findings from a representative Massachusetts high school sample. *American Journal of Health, 101*, 1683–1689. https://doi.org/10.2105/AJPH.2011.300155
51. Carabez, R., Pellegrini, M., Mankovitz, A., Eliason, M., & Scott, M. (2015). "never in all my years....": Nurses' education about LGBT health. *Journal of Professional Nursing, 31*(4), 323–329. https://doi.org/10.1016/j.profnurs.2015.01.003

52. Day, J. K., Fish, J. N., Perez-Brumer, A., Hatzenbuehler, M. L., & Russell, S. T. (2017). Transgender youth substance use disparities: Results from a population-based sample. *The Journal of Adolescent Health, 61*(6), 729–735. https://doi.org/10.1016/j.jadohealth.2017.06.024

53. Namaste, V. (2000). *Invisible lives: The erasure of transsexual and transgendered people.* University of Chicago Press.

54. Roller, C. G., Sedlak, C., & Drauker, C. B. (2015). Navigating the system: How transgender individuals engage in health care services. *Journal of Nursing Scholarship, 47*(5), 417–424. https://doi.org/10.1111/jnu.12160

55. Connell, R. W. (1987). *Gender and power: Society, the person and sexual politics.* Stanford University Press.

56. Connell, R. W. (2009). *Gender: In world perspective* (2nd ed.). Polity. https://doi.org/10.1177/0891243208327175

57. Link, B. G., & Phelan, J. C. (1996). Understanding socio-demographic differences in health— the role of fundamental social causes. *American Journal of Public Health, 86*(4), 471–473. https://doi.org/10.2105/AJPH.86.4.471

58. McPhail, D., Rountree-James, M., & Whetter, I. (2016). Addressing gaps in physician knowledge regarding transgender health and healthcare through medical education. *Canadian Medical Education Journal, 7*(2), e70–e78.

59. Poteat, T., German, D., & Kerrigan, D. (2013). Managing uncertainty: A grounded theory of stigma in transgender health care encounters. *Social Science & Medicine, 84*, 22–29. https://doi.org/10.1016/j.socscimed.2013.02.019

60. Sawning, S., Steinbock, S., Croley, R., Combs, R., Shaw, A., & Ganzel, T. (2017). A first step in addressing medical education curriculum gaps in lesbian, gay, bisexual, and transgender-related content: The University of Louisville Lesbian, gay, bisexual, and transgender health certificate program. *Education for Health, 30*(2), 108–114. https://doi.org/10.4103/efh.EfH_78_16

61. Buchholz, L. (2015). Transgender care moves into the mainstream. *Journal of the American Medical Association, 314*(17), 1785–1787. https://doi.org/10.1001/jama.2015.11043

62. McKay, B. (2011). Lesbian, gay, bisexual, and transgender health issues, disparities, and information resources. *Medical Reference Services Quarterly, 30*(4), 393–401. https://doi.org/10.1080/02763869.2011.608971

63. Khalili, J., Leung, L. B., & Diamont, A. (2015). Finding the perfect doctor: Identify lesbian, gay, bisexual, and transgender-competent physicians. *American Journal of Public Health, 105*(6), 1114–1119. https://doi.org/10.2105/AJPH.2014.302448

64. Baral, S. D., Beyrer, C., & Poteat, T. (2011). *Human rights, the law, and HIV among transgender people.* United Nations Development Programme, Bureau for Development Policy, HIV, Health & Development Group. http://www.hivlawcommission.org/index.php/working-papers?task+document.viewdoc&id=93

Tukea L. Talbert, D.N.P., R.N., C.D.P. is the Chief Diversity Officer for the University of Kentucky HealthCare System. As part of this role, she focuses on health equity for minoritized patient populations, which includes the LGBT (lesbian, gay, bisexual, and transgender) patients. Her key areas of focus include expanding the health equity data infrastructure to demographic and sexual orientation and gender identity (SOGI) analyses with health outcomes; optimization of the electronic health record to capture sexual orientation and gender identity (SOGI), pronouns, and preferred names of all patients; execution of best practices as outlined by the Healthcare Equality Index (HEI).

Part III
Cultural Models that Address
Quality of Care

Chapter 8
Brown Bodies in Pain and the Call for Narrative Medicine

Monica D. Griffin

Pain, as "the most common reason for seeking healthcare in the Western world" [1], warrants critical attention among healthcare providers in order to deliver culturally responsive care. Adequate care for pain remains elusive for healthcare providers, especially given the wide range of possibilities for its cause in patients. Differentiated treatment for pain is well-documented in Emergency Departments (EDs), but many studies fail to delve far enough into the pain patients experience and process for managing treatment to sustain effective outcomes. Diagnostic, therapeutic, surgical, and often pharmaceutical approaches dominate in a biomedical industry that treats pain largely as a quantifiable medical phenomena, measured and indicated through technoscientific procedures. O'Mahony [2]. urges narrative medicine scholars to teach the theory and practice of narratology toward two goals: (1) offering medical students "a connection with broader culture, a connection with the world beyond the medical school and the hospital" and (2) "an understanding of the place of medicine in society, the historical forces that have shaped it, and the challenges it will face in the future" (7). US medicine and health policymakers are currently confronted by the challenge of an opioid epidemic in conflation with pain management, and now the disparate comorbidities associated with the COVID-19 pandemic, with limited understanding of the pain patient's experience of treatment [3]. In this chapter, the author challenges social assumptions about cultural difference and systemic racism, in a qualitative, narrative medicine exploration of race and pain in brown-bodied patients.

Kalitzkus and Matthiessen [4]. describe four (4) genres of narrative medicine, the methodologies for which can advance toward more utilitarian goals of the

M. D. Griffin (✉)
Charles Center, William and Mary, Williamsburg, VA, USA
e-mail: mdgrif@wm.edu

R. Scales, A. T. McCleary-Gaddy (eds.), *Cultural Issues in Healthcare*,
https://doi.org/10.1007/978-3-031-20826-3_8

scholarship, as advocated by O'Mahony [2]: (1) patient stories—classic illness narratives; (2) physicians' stories; (3) narratives about physician-patient encounters; and (4) grand stories—e.g., metanarratives (sociocultural understanding of the body in health and illness). The authors state that "[n]arratives about being ill and caring for the ill provide insight into respective experience and thus could foster mutual understanding…" (2). Furthermore, "[n]arratives—especially patient narratives—incorporate the question of causality and thus foster an understanding of the patient's illness perception," which is itself determined by a chronology of encounters and treatments, and can impact the success of treatment and healing (1). This chapter's author uses an autobiographical narrative about her experience of chronic pain to reveal a uniquely female and brown-bodied experience of pain through the journey of treatment for it. The following chapter attempts to cover multiple perspectives for the treatment of chronic pain, with admittedly limited insight into the physician's perspective. However, the implications for care are highlighted where relevant in order to suggest that "narrative medicine" offers multiple methodologies for providers to establish greater rapport with their patients in comanaging more effective treatments.

I Am African American

I was not prepared for the journey that began with an emergency C-section and the healthy birth of a nearly nine-pound baby. This would be the third abdominal surgery of what would be four in the making of a journey of years of chronic pain; she was the first and only birth-child, in a complicated lifestyle with a driven work ethic and a blended family. In a semi-conscious haze of triage, I remember whispering to a set of nurses who hovered over me in their concern that my abdomen continued to swell after birth: "I am African American." They were fretting aloud over what to do now that the doctor had rushed away from his 3-day long shift to the comfort of a home shower at the unfortunate time that my body decided to hemorrhage internally. However, this story was going to end, I wanted them to get it right, both for me and my child: "I am African American."

Centering the Brown-Bodied Patient's Experience

What it means to be a brown-bodied person in a medical setting is rift with the complexity of what it means to be so in any social setting, except that the medical setting presents a peculiar set of tense circumstances for understanding a person's body and illness. Furthermore, social class, education, citizen status, and various other cultural factors significantly determine a patient's access to, compliance with, and use of resources in navigating a health experience within the medical system. The impact of daily stress, due to ongoing racism in addition to political and economic oppression on brown-bodied people[1] in the US potentially compounds the social

---

[1] Hereinafter, the author will refer to people of color as brown-bodied persons.

psychological experience of seeking and receiving care, in addition to reifying the already existent health disparities between racial and ethnic populations in North America.

For the purposes of this chapter, the term "brown bodies" refers to a broad population of human beings whose bodies are encased within brown-hued skin, regardless of nationality, preferred or ascribed racial identity, or genealogy. Although much of this chapter's analysis is based on the experiences and data of African Americans (in direct relation to the identity of the author/autoethnographer), the term is used here intentionally to encompass a vast range of sociohistorical experiences of people of color throughout the globe. Variation across the range of sociohistorical experiences referenced here are not medically irrelevant; however, the author aims to capture the uniquely North American cultural experience that fixates on skin tone in determining situational relationships. Because the North American experience historically and conceptually engages race as a cultural matter of skin tone, the author presupposes that the clinical pain management in US healthcare is largely invariant across brown-bodied patients, except in obvious cases of specific racism, or during periods of heightened and specified geo-sociopolitical tension.

Barbara Fields and Karen Fields [5] argue persuasively that the popular, political, and sometimes social scientific collapsing of racial groups (defined loosely in terms of ancestry or geography—as in, country of origin) can have the effect of minimizing the impact of social class, religion, and other important aspects of social experience and life as significantly interrelated. According to the Fields, it is a fictional practice they term "racecraft" in scholarship and everyday life to understand race as uniformly experienced within prescribed categories of existence that are soundly refuted by biological and anthropological research in the last half-century. Furthermore, the Fields argue, emphasis on race grouping for its own sake, mistakenly places focus on individuals as explanations for how they are treated, instead of identifying the racist or race-based behaviors of others and the structural, institutional factors at work. The goal of this chapter is not to counter or refute that important work but instead focuses on the *socially* constructed nature of race as it is also located in the *social psychology* of one brown-bodied patient, in order to examine the merits of a strategy for centering the patient's narrative of illness in investigating pain treatment. It is not offered here as a methodology for generalizing health outcomes according to race categories.

Increasingly corporatized, medical institutions have turned toward cultural competence or diversity training approaches to addressing racism and other forms of bias in healthcare. Others have suggested more community-based, integrative approaches to diversity in the form of cultural humility, which centers the experience of the individual in question as a significant source of knowledge in developing care and treatment plans for patients [6]. Gravlee's [7] scholarship on "how race becomes biology" explores racial inequality in health in order to "refine the critique of race" (e.g., underscoring the concept's inconsistency with patterns of global human genetic diversity, refocusing attention on environmental and life-course influences on health). Gravlee recommends that scholars "expand research on the sociocultural reality of race and racism" in order to better understand the interconnection between biological and physiological phenomenon with social and cultural. The present research elaborates a conception of "brown-bodied" pain as a strategy for understanding the *embodiment* of pain as a physiological and social psychological condition that is variously informed by a wide range of social determinants, many of which derive from lived, racialized experiences including, but not limited to racism. Through narrative medicine, the author hopes to illustrate ways that illness and pain are differentially embodied and mediated by racialized individuals in North American society. Although healthcare is invariably managed by a formalized, medical model of care, health disparities persist across demographic comparisons in ways that suggest the need for culturally responsive care that is richly informed by human experiences.

Sustaining Life Between ED and Home
Following the birth of my child, it would take at least 4 weeks of recovery to regain strength, just to walk and sit upright, let alone lift and feed my hefty baby girl. Her adoring stepsisters and dad faded into the background while my (full-time employed) mother and sisters took weekly shifts to assist with feeding and changing the baby; they took time off to do this in addition to feeding me and changing my own sheets, as fevers and night sweat sapped all my energy and focus. During this time, I returned twice to the Emergency Department (ED) with escalated blood pressure and a fever that sometimes indicated the possibility of infection. At other times, with differing rounds of ED doctors, it indicated my body's attempt to restabilize after having lost nearly enough blood for a transfusion. Her father and I rushed to create legal documents for her health care in the advent of my death, having learned that "they" had found the infection. I imagined a mysterious team of lab technicians peering nonchalantly into microscope at my anonymous, Emergency Department blood and urine samples until Eureka! They found it. Although no one ever said so, my medically straightforward history of endometriosis, coupled with my cervix's failure to dilate probably complicated the birth, and led to this very real concern: I could die. I was given antibiotics, pain medications, and less sodium in my diet, and I was hesitantly reassured that I might survive to see my child grow up. I remember looking back at my daughter's small head of hair nestled safely in my own mother's arms, whispering a frightened goodbye each time more desperately than the prior exodus to the ED. I contemplated whether I would live to raise my "miracle" baby, having endured 4 years of treated infertility.

So much for Black women's fecundity! I had evaded the stereotype of black teenage pregnancy, bolstered by insistent cautions and warnings from a host of aunts and older cousins in my family as the end of many women's dreams, a shame on the community. (Not that I believed it then or now; but I did live amidst it.) Instead, I had waited, through a couple of marriages, advanced degrees, and a mortgage to reach a barrier within my own body; my own female body betrayed me! Without bearing children, was I still woman? And still, after years of treatment, my child's arrival now signaled the literal end of my own life? Had I made a critical error against nature—investing time, hope, and money in creating a human being who would live without her mother?

Rita Charon [8] describes four different kinds of divides between the sick and the healthy—divisions which emerge in a patient's telling of their story as indicative of differences between a patient's and a provider's perspective of illness:

1. *The relation to mortality*, in which doctors relate materially to mortality, as an accepted part of the human body; whereas, patients view death as both "unthinkable and inevitable";
2. *The contexts of illness,* in which doctors consider illness in terms of biological events with technically discernable causes; whereas, patients consider illness in the "frame and scope" of their entire lives;
3. *Beliefs about disease causality,* wherein beliefs about causality can dictate action, and healthcare providers can ascribe meanings to illness, which influence treatment, action, and sometimes conflicting views with patients;
4. *The emotions of shame, blame, and fear,* which exist as frequently undisclosed factors in the experience of illness and care, yet have an immeasurably powerful impact on suffering for either care provider or patient (22).

The author's vignettes above demonstrate each of these divisions, to some degree.

Another goal of this research is to center the brown-bodied patient's experience of healthcare, especially since care is not limited to medical settings for immediate and appropriate response. A child's birth story, for example, constitutes the beginning of the author's conscious journey with chronic pain, because it registers a series of related events within the archives of medical records across several clinics and organizations of care. From infertility to the diagnosis of endometriosis to sciatic pain during pregnancy to a complicated emergency delivery that resulted in hemorrhaging and postnatal infection, the drama escalates in ways that may appear to be standard to healthcare providers across OB/Gyn as well as Reproductive Health specialists and Endocrinologists. But Maternal Health providers know differently, that the experience *is* more complicated than the technical aspects of labor and illness; childbirth is family embedded, and part of a larger emotional and cultural reality. Said one ED nurse during a follow-up emergency visit: "You're the kind of patient that is why I got out of Maternity Care. Hope and fear all mixed up together for the whole family, and then this. It's awful. Baby's okay, though, right? And now, you're here. You made it past delivery, though. Hang in there."

Friends, family, spouses, lovers, and children share in a person's life outside of the institutional backdrop of a clinic or an ED. They retain information and influence a person's experiences and behaviors through managing medication, assisting with therapies, and mediating compliance and noncompliance—often in ways that are not known by clinical providers. "She can't sit up long enough to feed her," my sister whispered into the phone to a lactation counselor so I would not hear her, then gently handed me the phone so the counselor could talk me through a decision to feed by bottle. She suggested this way I could focus on my healing and enjoy my child's satisfaction in being fed. A patient's "story" arguably constitutes a network of actions, communications, and care that extends beyond site-based clinical encounters, yet this network and these intimate, infinite experiences bear on the health of the patient immeasurably. How a patient internalizes and then engages in the process of health crisis or healing encompasses many factors, including psychological mechanisms of comprehension and understanding, spiritual beliefs, subjective feelings, and personal biases. The so-called personal, patient realities that are often deemed irrelevant aspects of a health experience, come unavoidably into contact with the technical, medical, and similarly subjective realities of (usually healthy) other people in mediating healthcare. This chapter explores an autobiographic narrative of illness, as informed by and contextualized within a life history, which itself is contextualized by a racialized history of medical practice in science and healthcare.

Brown-Bodied Encounters in Medical Settings: From the Past to the Present

Social encounters between healthcare providers and brown bodies is an important opportunity to improve healthcare treatment practices, but the chasms between standardized treatment protocols for variant causes of illness (pain, for example) are further compounded by the challenge of culturally responsive treatment. No one social group, or life history, can be over-simplified or—generalized when considering the range of factors that impact any individual's experience of pain management, for example. Some brown-bodied social histories are additionally embedded within systems of violence and oppression and further compounded by gender, beliefs, lack of wealth, knowledge, and family relationships. All of these factors permeate the human experience of medical settings and can be further complicated in the brown-bodied person's social encounter with medical professionals. Because brown-bodied patients are more likely to see doctors whose physiognomy, or race and ethnicity, is different than their own, their cultural values, norms, and beliefs may also be different. The chasm between the healthy and the sick, described by Charon above, both situates and intensifies the complexity of treating brown-bodied patients and for their experience of care.

My Big, Brown-ish, Happy Family

Before my child's birth, my mostly brown-bodied family filled the Maternity Ward's waiting room easily, spilling into the hallway to get food, play games, contribute their baby welcome messages to a "home" video in-the-making. Some of them encouraged the baby to "Hurry up!" so they could teach her who she (or he) was, in family and cultural terms. They passed the time recalling other family birth stories and cooing over my 10-month-old niece. In-laws, grandparents, friends, and immediate family comprised nearly 15 people spanning European, Cuban, Puerto Rican, and African American ancestries in the ward for an entire Saturday from 7 a.m. when I was induced until 10:51 p.m. when she was born. They joked later how they "took over" the ward with their food, their music, and mostly loud conversation. They celebrated their social and cultural difference in this context, later boasting to one another how they had transformed this highly "medical" space into "their family space." Most came from a neighboring city, but others traveled several hours and across states to be present. We had prayed and waited a very long time for this tiny person. Years later, when my daughter and I would regularly watch the video of her first bath, being weighed, and then laid in a crib for the family to see her, we would often marvel at the size of the crowd of family in the window peering and pointing at her. In-law grandparents commented in playful awe and competition about how much she looks like "their son" or "their daughter." My daughter has often remarked, "It's amazing how loved I was before I was ever really known."

But they did know her. For them, she was the culminating victory of prayers for a child, costly and emotionally draining infertility treatments, a discontinued (despite thousands of dollars invested) adoption process, and the miracle of a more relaxed, Ph.D. professional woman in their family who had conceived naturally after quitting a tenured job in academia. The family had collectively pitched in to help a newly unemployable pregnant professional with food and paid for prenatal healthcare out-of-pocket until a transition to new insurance coverage could be made. In private contrast to my daughter's remark, family members have reflected darkly that at this very time of joy, I was in another room "fighting" to live. Their acknowledgment of this contrast, in their memory and telling of the story, is not merely one of irony; it is part of the spiritual journey—this was all meant to be however fragile and mysterious the reality of life was.

Interactions between healthcare providers and patients can range from single encounters (as in an Emergency Department) to short-term physical therapy and long-term relationships (as in the case of chronic pain or illness). Treatment for pain in brown bodies has varied across time and region, identity and nationality, diagnoses and life chances, changes, and choices. Specialized education and generally higher social class of medical doctors typically stand in contrast to the predominantly lower income and moderate education levels of most brown-bodied patients. Even when brown-bodied patients encounter providers with a similar social class, depending on the practitioner's role or the patient's social class, the encounter is almost certainly accompanied by a set of assumptions about behavioral norms (such as what modes of transportation a person uses, affordability of medication, flexibility of job release for continuing therapies, etc.). Sometimes the assumptions lead to racism, miscommunication, and mutual misunderstanding.

Brown-Bodied Narratives: Finding the Illness Is Part of the Story, Past and Present

Behind every brown-bodied individual who requires pain assessment, diagnosis, treatment, and pain management is a social history. An inexhaustible number of personal and situational factors mold the contours of that social history, which is itself embedded in a broader context of historical and cultural factors that inform their beliefs, interaction, fears, decisions, and actions related to illness and recovery. North American medicine's treatment of African Americans is a historically dismal starting point for considering brown-bodied cultural assumptions related to medical research, practice, and treatment. Arguably, not all brown-bodied individuals in the United States actually know and recall details of this history or attribute it to their own identities (and therefore perceptions about social interactions in medicine as racialized). But even cursory knowledge, however accurate or mythical, serves to feed a general narrative and culture of distrust, drawing on just a sample of widely known violations in ethical practice involving persons of African descent in North America.

Harriet A. Washington [9] outlines a time continuum of the relationship between North American medicine and brown bodies, particularly African Americans, in the well-known anthology, *Medical Apartheid: the Dark History of Medical Experimentation on Black Americans from Colonial Times to the Present*. Washington describes medical uses and abuses of brown bodies, including examples from exploitative experimentation and voyeurism—a ghastly trail of unethical and exploitative clinical malpractices in which practitioners treated (in this case, black) bodies inhumanely toward research on disease progression and response to treatment. Most prominently known among these is perhaps the Tuskegee Syphilis Experiment, a case in which physicians injected African American men with placebo treatment for syphilis, without their knowledge or consent, in order to observe the progression of infection in their bodies. Most egregious in this case was the continuation of this practice even after the discovery of Penicillin as a cure to relieve symptoms. President Bill Clinton's (1997) apology for the abuse of human rights and medical ethics in the Tuskegee Experiment is noted as one of the first of its kind [10]. Another more recent case involves the case of Henrietta Lacks, whose unique cells were retrieved during an excruciatingly painful trial of cancer, without her unquestionable consent or knowledge, and used (by an entire industry of medical research) for the scientific development of cures to a number of illnesses—and as social pattern would have it, without attribution, communication, or compensation to her surviving family, many of whom would not have known or would not have had the resources to benefit from said discoveries [11]. Subjugation to research and experimentation preyed particularly on the economically vulnerable, persons whose social origins were subSaharan African, as well as youth populations.

Washington details the guiding role of North American medicine in the Eugenics Movement globally, and the persistent biological and molecular bias that situates brown bodies perversely in comparison to animals as inferior, apart from a ranging continuum of humans, even in the face of evidence disputing essentialist arguments about race.[2] Importantly, Washington's work forms a foundational understanding of longstanding institutional abuse on the part of North American medicine that forms the basis and culturally persistent distrust of doctors, the system, and society, on the part of African Americans, even in the maintenance of their well-being.

---

[2] See the Washington [9] text for detailed information about the Tuskegee Experiment, circus animus shows, the miraculous Henrietta Lacks cells, and others, for examples. Also, other chapters within this textbook address other examples of social factors that impact medical treatment for minorities.

For example, Keith Wailoo [12] studies the evolution of medical research and treatment for sickle cell anemia as "an authentic Black disease" from invisibility to visibility, in public consciousness as much as medical practice. He writes in *Dying in the City of the Blues: Sickle Cell Anemia and the Politics of Race and Health (2014)*:

> Viewing the historical evolution of sickle cell anemia, we witness a series of shifts in which clinicians and scientists, patients and communities, politicians and movie actors, and society at large come to reinterpret and give fresh meanings to pain, blood cells, and disease experience (4).

Wailoo's scholarship connects the importance of understanding multiple viewpoints about the treatment of the disease itself, not merely for the purpose of forming a precise cellular understanding of the disorder and its prevalence but also for creating a broader understanding of pain treatment and disease politics in US healthcare.

African Americans are disproportionately identified as drug seekers in ED visits, compared to white persons, and are therefore less likely to be given opioid prescriptions for pain [13] during visits; consequently, they are more likely to be put at risk for the exacerbating impact of sustaining pain without treatment. Stang et al. [1] found in their metastudy of quality indicators in the assessment of pain in the ED, for example, continuing disparities in how medical professionals treat patients for pain:

> although opioid prescribing in the United States for patients with a pain-related ED visit increased after national quality improvements efforts in the 1990s, differences according to race and ethnicity have not dimished (31).... Other identified factors associated with delays in analgesia that deserve further exploration included language barriers (46) and insurance status (Medicaid) (40). Delays in analgesia were also more likely among children (69) and elderly patients (40, 69).

Social processes for navigating pain management, in particular, are both personal and social, comprised of acute and often continuing relationships that mediate an individual's treatment and, when possible, recovery. Pain management engages patients in encounters with healthcare providers—ranging from doctors to nurses, physician's assistants, and physical therapists—and each is likely to be found in any of a variety of medical settings and facilities. The doctors, nurses, and other personnel located within EDs are even further removed from patients' experiences, given their station within what can be considered a biomedical vortex of practice, communication, and social processes between clinical and medical institutions of all kinds, including pharmaceutical and insurance companies, employer institutions, and families. The ED is situated functionally as an organizational clearinghouse for sending acute as well as chronic pain patients to other clinical settings, if needed, for continuing care. In this function, the ED is an acute site for social transformation in mediating healthcare, with the potential to launch new, productive relationships between other clinical providers and patients. It is, in many cases, the first encounter in an individual's pain treatment or management, a service with which it is continually engaged; it is more likely than not, an intermediate space between diagnoses that formulate individualized pathologies of pain for individuals.

Advancements in technological evaluation and tools do not, on their own, advance doctors' and nurses' ability to definitively diagnose pain. Singhal et al. [13] use the following examples for characterizing conditions of pain as coded within EDs:

> Non-definitive conditions: using primary reason for visit coding, (1) toothache, back pain, and abdominal pain;
>   Definitive conditions: using the primary diagnosis, such as long-bone fractures and kidney stones.

[Note: the inherent definition of "definitive" in the study relies on the presence of diagnostic technologies that are willingly performed and can affirm the condition with a high amount of scientific certainty, as in imaging.] The study's findings reveal that a greater proportion of non-definitive conditions are presented in visits to the ED by racial-ethnic minorities and younger adults; only 27–47% of ED visits were made by patients with private insurance, where the majority were either uninsured or Medicaid beneficiaries; and compared to patients with definitive conditions, a greater proportion of patients with non-definitive conditions had repeatedly visited the ED in the past year. "Non-Hispanic blacks had significantly lower odds…of receiving opioids during their ED visits for back pain and abdominal pain compared to non-Hispanic whites. However, no racial-ethnic differences in opioid administration were found among ED visits for toothache, and the definitive conditions" (4).[3]

Racial-ethnic minority patients, especially non-Hispanic blacks presenting with vague conditions often associated with drug-seeking behavior, may be more likely to be judged as a "drug-seeker" relative to a non-Hispanic white patient, presenting with similar pain-related complaints. This is especially concerning [Singhal et al. note] in light of a recent study that found that the prevalence of opioid abuse and addiction is lower among Hispanics and non-Hispanic Blacks, compared to non-Hispanic whites [14].

When and How Did the Pain Start?

That's a question commonly asked by medical professionals and practitioners who treat pain as the most prevalent symptom of an array of medical issues. The birth of my child is my earliest memory of postpartum sciatic pain. Sciatica had started during my pregnancy and got worse, following the C-Section and recovery. I began working 10 months after giving birth, as an instructor-professional in higher education and public health. I had "good insurance" with resources to see as many orthopedic specialists, rehabilitative physicians, chiropractors, and trainers as my schedule could hold. I could get X-rays, MRIs, CT scans, and bone density scans as

---

[3] Singhal et al. [13] acknowledge a number of limitations with their study, including variability in clinical presentation of pain and its severity, the degree to which a non-definitive classification for presentation of pain (such as abdominal) can be associated with a definitive classification (such as pancreatitis) serves to underestimate disparities, and others, but argue nonetheless, that they demonstrate significant racial-ethnic disparities in opioid prescription and administration in ED visits for non-definitive conditions. Physicians' humanity enjoins knowledge and skill with judgment in multiple contexts of diagnosis and biases that encumber an authority-endowed role's capacity to offer effective and humane treatment.

long as they weren't too much at one time for my body to contain radiation. Over that extended period of time, I took medication that controlled the endometriosis but compromised my bone density in the end. I followed all the instructions—to eat certain foods, exercise regularly, keep the weight down—except one: don't pick up the heavy, growing toddler. I fell in love with pilates, the only exercise my body seemed capable of doing without compromising my ability to walk and work—and raise two teens and a toddler. I managed what appeared to be a seemingly common circumstance for postpartum women—compromised hip structure, lingering back pain, and the mandate to fix myself by fixing my health behavior. Absent a glaring image or test, the road to recovery began with me and my behavior.

Ten years passed before my OB/Gyn finally agreed with my primary physician, chiropractor, massage therapist, and physical therapists: it was time for a hysterectomy. She held one final conversation with me about my certainty in not wanting to conceive again. I was incredulous that this had to be such a "careful" decision based on my desire to be a mother, and not necessarily based on my quality of life. Years of birth control medicines and Lupron injections (which I now understand is sometimes used to treat cancer) had reached their limit on compromising my bone density; pilates had become near impossible, and I was missing work for three full days every month in near perfect correlation with menstruation. A hysterectomy was sure to identify and cure the culprit: endometriosis. What followed this fourth abdominal surgery was severe disconnectivity between my pelvic muscles and the revelation of symptoms for what they were, just symptoms. The surgery determined that my endometriosis was in fact minimal, but I did have a condition known as "menstrual reflux" which was known to cause inflammation and pain. But instead of improving after the surgery, my pain worsened over the months that followed and my trips to the ED continued.

I learned that there is no real "pathology of pain" class for emergency room doctors. Never mind in a single year before the surgery, I had lost my mother, separated from my husband, developed kidney stones, suffered a nerve sprain in one foot, and developed a strange overload of allergies and asthma out of nowhere. What the Emergency Department saw in the six to eight visits during that period of time, was a black woman without a pain specialist. ED doctors also had limited patience for being ineffective dispensaries of medicine, instead of life-savers (which I suppose drew them to the field). I came to know variability in health care, despite persistence with ineffectively treated pain, through repeated encounters with sometimes the same doctor during my ED experiences. And despite well-integrated information systems, each visit detailing my surgical history, pain locations and medications, and elevated blood pressure—no one was assigned to the tracing the pain story, evaluating my symptoms as credible, or make their effort, intentions, or skills known to me for finding stability in health. Each time I was discharged with little to no more information than I had in the crisis-based visit before the last. How did this journey, which included an elaborate system of actors—skilled experts at treating the human body—always start and stop with me? With my knowledge and behavior alone?

The Biomedical TechnoService Complex, Inc.: An Elaborate Set of Actors

Biomedical TechnoService Complex, Inc. refers to increasingly corporatized and privatized modes of research, products, and services made available in medicine, a referent to Eisenhower's 1950s phrase about the dominance and size of US military organization. Clarke et al. [15] identify the following, most notable socioeconomic changes as indicative of, and facilitating biomedicalization: (1) corporatization and commodification; (2) centralization, rationalization, and devolution of services; and (3) stratified biomedicalization. "Biomedicalization" theory describes a complex set of social transformations that has fundamentally altered the field of medicine as an industry based on market forces, emergent technologies, and evolving social bodies and identities. In the context of the Biomedical TechnoService Complex, Inc., brown-bodied persons disproportionately have had to navigate torrential waves through political and practical gauntlets to receive quality healthcare, admittedly alongside others.

Clarke et al. characterize biomedicalization processes as "situated within a dynamic and expanding politico-economic and sociocultural biomedical sector… reciprocally constituted and manifested through five major interactive processes":

1. the politico-economic constitution of the Biomedical TechnoService Complex, Inc. [the originating authors' term];
2. the focus on health itself and elaboration of risk and surveillance biomedicine;
3. the increasingly technoscientific nature of the practices and innovations of biomedicine;
4. transformations of biomedical knowledge production, information management, distribution, and consumption; and,
5. transformations of bodies to include new properties and the production of new individual and collective technoscientific identities.

Biomedical, social, and institutional processes in US medicine are not mutually exclusive, in that they transform and reconstitute one another in various ways over time. Brown-bodied persons experience the impact of biomedical social transformation in sometimes common, but often distinctive ways that deserve some understanding as a context for the population's experience of pain and illness.

According to 2015 data from the US Department of Health and Human Services, Office of Minority Health, "54.4% of non-Hispanic blacks in comparison to 75.8% of non-Hispanic whites used private health insurance. Also in 2015, 43.6% of non-Hispanic blacks in comparison to 32.7% of non-Hispanic whites relied on Medicaid, public health insurance. Finally, 11.0% of non-Hispanic blacks in comparison to 6.3% of non-Hispanic whites were uninsured."[4] Recent research indicates, too, that immigrant and refugee populations may experience a higher prevalence of health

---

[4] https://minorityhealth.hhs.gov/omh/browse.aspx?lvl=3&lvlid=61; last accessed 1/29/17.

conditions due to limited access to healthcare and insurance coverage over the span of time-related to their status and settlement in the United States [16].

Biomedicalization provides an important context for understanding the complicated, often interconnected experiences of brown bodies in health, especially the experiences of individuals who live with chronic pain. The social transformations and co-constitutive processes of North American medicine correlate with broader social, economic, and political phenomena that racialize populations as brown-bodied individuals, subjugating them to discriminatory treatment. However, biomedicalization is an emergent social transformation with the capacity for adaptation and interventions that could democratize healthcare delivery and sustained treatment. Clarke et al. suggest, in fact, that "the increasingly complex, multi-sited, multidirectional processes of medicalization… today are being both extended and reconstituted through the emergent social forms and practices of a highly and increasingly technoscientific biomedicine." With biomedicalization has come a shift in the processes by which clinics collect and communicate information one that is increasingly technical, led by emerging new technologies for evaluating, treating, intervening, and promoting health and better health outcomes, on one hand. As innovations continue at a rapid pace, it has exposed new opportunities, on the other hand, to reimagine how medical departments or clinics collect and use information, such as that which is possible through narrative medicine.

Get Yourself a Pain Doctor

In one of my early visits, one doctor heaped upon me mounds of advice about heating pads, lidocaine patches, the need for regular exercise, ointments, and even asked to pray over me (through my "Level 9" pain). (No manner of eloquence in explaining my health journey of pain, therapies, and medication that led to a hysterectomy and increased pain and disability, could dissuade her from teaching—maybe preaching?—that my behavior, above all, would cure the pain.) On another visit, she gave me direct, coherent advice with a powerful narcotic prescription: "Get a pain doctor—they mediate all this medication in a way that will treat you faster than all these other specialists can." At last, she could see my intense search for care in the computer's medical history. (I think I actually told her to look!) I carried that advice straight to a recommended pain specialist, but not in time to evade another pain crisis. In the last encounter with this particular doctor, I believe that inflammation in my spine and pelvic region had reached the point of compressing my pudendal nerves causing bladder spasms that did not allow me to void urine. It must have been a strange night; she had forgotten who I was—her patient. Yes, I was a repeat visitor. Yes, I always required powerful pain medication as a response. But, hadn't we reached a common understanding that I needed help during my last visit? Hadn't she pulled up the same set of charts, and details on her computer? While I writhed in pain, during the time I had assumed it was taking for an army of medical staff to be sure I was not drug-seeking by reading my chart, she abandoned our doctor–patient relationship as one of mutual trust and responsibility. Instead, I overheard her talking in another drape-partitioned room, "Everybody's crying tonight and there's nothing I can do. 'I can't pee! I need meds!' What the heck!" In my mind, I had ceased being a human adult to her. I was no longer a human being who needed a compassionate response and reassurance that my bladder would not rupture internally, putting me at severe risk of septic infection. My mother passed away due to MRSA infection, inside an Emergency Department that had two decades prior saved her life from cardiac arrest. Hadn't I told her that? Didn't she understand why I would be freaking out? Life and death, and all that?

Of course, it occurred to me over and over again, despite having a light brown complexion: was I too brown to have legitimate pain? Had I mistakenly worn a #blacklivesmatter T-shirt into the ED? I recalled all the seemingly friendly conversations I had with doctors, nurses, and the myriad others in the ED team: I teach health disparities. Did they imagine this as some elaborate experiment to see if I could play the system for medication? Prove them faulty? The dear friend who accompanied me to the ED that night had suggested that I let the doctors do the searching, and stop being so calm and precise in my descriptions of what was happening. Maybe then they would hear me, see me, treat me. I tried the patient role from a different place of need, indeed a desperate one. I let myself scream when the doctor pressed against my foot and into my hip. I cried incessantly as the pain was incessant, and I breathed and groaned like a woman in labor with each spasm. I was genuinely confused: I had no more uterus, and until this night, had no idea that bladders could spasm. Furious at hearing my report of the doctor's comment—one that broke my spirit and sent me into desperate requests that he handle my affairs if needed, he held my hand tightly through waves of excruciating, physiologically ineffective bladder spasms and finally whispered into my ear: "If it can come out at all, just piss all over this *expletive* bed. Jeez!" Finally, in addition to pain medication, I had to get an emergency catheter to release over a L of urine, which was then taped to my leg for referral to a urologist. It could not be removed for over a week, during which time it was entirely up to me if I wanted to slosh to and from work, to empty urine, and sustain hygiene in a public bathroom. (I understood the medical need for catheters. Keep in mind, my condition was pain. What would the "doctor's note" say if stayed home? What could it say if I went to work?) By then a single mother of a teenager, I spent a week in bed, waiting out the spasms until an appointment became available for a different specialty's round of diagnostics.

Healthcare providers' roles as evaluators of pain nonetheless remain pivotal in mediating health outcomes, despite technological innovation to diagnose illness and treat it. In the case of pain, those innovations remain limited, while patterns in ED evaluations of pain suggest the need to change how healthcare providers profile patients in assessing pain. Non-vigilant treatment outcomes are not good for anyone; untreated, chronic pain results in return visits and sometimes comorbidities that necessitate the prescription of opioid medications. But North American patient surveillance need not be limited to tracking technical information and sharing between medical clinics and settings; it could be attentive, diagnostic, and used extensively as a baseline that informs a larger story of the patient's experience of illness. Currently, clinical prejudice or doctor-driven racialized profiling for care *is* the practice, as a matter of cultural, as much as institutional practice—in documented empirical patterns of contemporary medicine as much as historical. Although biomedical industries may appear to be maximizing bureaucratic efficiency in correspondence with pharmaceutical and insurance market forces regarding patients' healthcare, healthcare delivery has become a commodity that ultimately devalues humanity in human conditions, especially those found in brown bodies, when viewed and treated through the lenses of professional biases, dismissive and discriminatory practices of meting out treatments.

Narrative Medicine: What It Can and Cannot Offer

Rita Charon [8] suggests "that what medicine lacks today—in singularity, humility, accountability, empathy—can, in part, be provided through intensive narrative training. Literary studies and narrative theory, on the other hand, seek practical ways to transduce their conceptual knowledge into palpable influence in the world, and a connection with health care can do that" (p. viii). Narrative medicine at its best is an "interdisciplinary, process-based approach to examine suffering, illness, disability, personhood, therapeutic relationships, and meaning in health care [18] One example of its positive impact on healthcare is seen in the differences between children's hospitals and other facilities for general health care. "Along with their growing scientific expertise, doctors need the expertise to listen to their patients, to understand as best they can the ordeals of illness, to honor the meanings of their patients' narratives of illness, and to be moved by what they behold so that they can act on their patients' behalf" (Charon, 3).

I Think You've Been Under-Diagnosed
It took more than 10 years, a laparoscopic surgery, partial hysterectomy, and at least eight visits to the ED the last of them, for an orthopedic surgeon (with residence experience in anomalies) to diagnose and name my condition: Bertolloti's Syndrome (BS—I find the acronym more amusing!). BS refers to a congenital, degenerative spinal anomaly in which the individual develops any one of several variations in the alignment and fusion of lumbosacral transitional vertebrae. ("See 2015 Landmark Study" [20] is a reference we use in the Facebook Group I use for most BS medical information, experiential and science-based, to denote our own classification type and concomitant patterns of pain, eligibility for surgical intervention, etc. We tell one another to carry copies of the study into new medical appointments with us since it will probably be needed.) The recently modified [17] Castellvi Classification System indicates precisely how vertebrae are differently fused, or not, to the sacral bone (which is sometimes not fully developed), causing inflammation, arthritis, overuse, malalignment, biomechanical dysfunctions, and pain. I know this because I studied this; 1 year before the publication of the "2015 Landmark Study" I took a medical leave to do the research myself in clinical trials that spanned EDs, rehabilitative doctors, OB/GYNs, urologists, neurologists, orthopedic surgeons, and primary care. I pulled every professional and family string I

could, to be seen by specialists outside my region and they pulled the same World Health Organization report on the condition that I had already read about on the Internet. It is not simply an SI Joint Dysfunction, Piriformis Syndrome, Lower Lumbar Pain, Degenerative Disc Disease, Arthritis, Bursitis, IT Band Syndrome, or any number of diagnostic codes that have been used to document the geography of my bodily pain symptoms—the narrative of diagnostic codes my new pain doctor began to produce while testing the effectiveness of injections in my spine and joints. It is BS, Bertolotti Syndrome, the hidden time bomb in my spine that torments some people in earlier ages and leaves others alone for the entirety of their lifetime. It could become progressively worse, it could improve with some behaviors I had begun. Before returning to work, I requested accommodations, requested handicap parking, and in arguing my case for it, had to pull up the X-Ray for my primary care physician to interpret the image. He commented after my explanation, "I think you've been underdiagnosed this whole time!"

Ironically, I remembered that one of the best orthopedists in my region, at the earliest point in my journey, had seen BS on an x-ray before when I first reported pain; but despite my repeated presentation with debilitating pain, he dismissed it as largely a mild condition (and in his view, more likely, it was just a variation in the way that doctors "counted lumbar"). Short periods of pain medication and longer periods of physical therapy would be enough, in his estimate. His colleague, a second ortho surgeon consult for me, said as much even a decade later. (I later learned online she was prolifically making a name for herself in the region, giving talks on the importance of discontinuing opioid medication. She refused to offer me any other treatment than the injection she had tried, which proved ineffective. (On this, we disagreed. To her, my leg's twitch indicated she was effective—at hitting the nerve or muscle—summarily dismissing my continuing pain and immobility as a relevant indicator of ineffectiveness). To my knowledge, this expert never consulted with my pain specialist who continued in the same vein, until I declined further injections from him. In a final visit for a piriformis injection, the "45 mins" I was assured that my leg's total paralysis would last, extended instead late into the evening. Concerned that my bladder might shut down again, I called for EMT support and requested a bladder ultrasound "based on my history" I explained to a befuddled ED team. "Yes, my urologist is in the other health network. Yes, they performed a voiding analysis. This is spinal; I have a neurogenic bladder related to diagnosed chronic pain in my spine." The ED team ED attempted to reach my pain specialist to no avail; once a friend picked me up in a wheelchair, and deposited me at home with dinner and assistance to the bathroom, his responsibility to me was done. When I assured the ED Team that I did want, in fact had brought my own with me, they did the scan to be sure nothing was happening that I could not feel. I slept in the ED until another friend could retrieve me at 6 a.m.

Arntfield et al. [18] studied the perceived influence of narrative medicine training on clinical skill development of 4th-year medical students. "Students explicitly linked the process and content of their learning to their perceived future effectiveness as physicians." In their study, the "utility of methods" of narrative methods are challenged and questions about "changes experienced as a result of training" arise. A review by Shapiro et al. notes that "many educational initiatives rooted in the humanities are limited in their capacity to succeed due to significant resistance posed by both students and faculty [46]." Obviously, doctors do not become doctors in order to tell or listen to stories. But the Arntfield et al. study shows that

> …[junior] residents identified their skill in story-telling and story-listening to be tools in the work of medicine itself. They recognized the centrality of story-telling in their daily interactions with peers, superiors, patients, and families. One found that the narrative interpretive skill allowed for culturally sensitive understanding of patients. The language itself is the critical narrative element—in writing notes and communicating to and about patients (284).

Studies on the practice of narrative medicine are predominantly focused on medical student assessments of its usefulness, but research on qualitative methods in collecting data, treating pain, and following up with patients with chronic conditions have yielded important results too.

Stang et al. [1] performed a metastudy on the use of quality indicators for the assessment of pain in the emergency department, in research conducted between 1980 and 2010. Since "inadequate pain treatment can have detrimental effects" such as "extended length of hospitalization, slower healing, altered pain processing, depression, anxiety, and substantial social and economic costs to society" and the individual, the authors demonstrate that previous research indicates improvement in the quality of care provided to patients and health outcomes, using quality indicators. Quality indicators that were studied included: "the count of indicators for the assessment and treatment of pain in the ED (including the type of indicator (structure [such as staff, equipment, and facilities], process [prescribing, investigations, interactions between professionals and patients], or outcome [such as mortality, morbidity or patient satisfaction]) and the aspect of pain measured (assessment or management)." Related to the earlier assertion of biomedicalization as a major context for understanding the necessity and feasibility of narrative medicine, the authors found that 80% (eighty percent) of pain studies in the ED focused on the care process, while 15% focused on structure. But only 5% focused on patient outcome.

The Pain Patient's Role

As a chronic pain patient, I remember a few doctors who showed consistent kindness or time in helping me face what would become a chronic lifestyle of managing pain, stigma, diminishing mobility, and ability, through what I like to think of as recidivist cycles of recovery. Nurses had more time with me, but they were prone to the screening demeanors of avoiding eye contact, and not assuming recognition or familiarity with a patient in a process of health recovery; afterall, brown-bodied recidivist ED visitors are easily labeled drug seekers. Only initially, in postpartum care, did nurses request return shifts and visit to see that I had survived. I learned within my brown skin, that it matters little how accurately one documents the physical reality they are experiencing, how much one uses the jargon of the field (such as telling them "I have 50 mg of Tramadol and 25 mg of Zipsor on board" when you want to avoid an overdose, despite the level of pain or escalating blood pressure indicator). It matters little that you have mastered breathing, to wait patiently without screaming while they take the tests they need, see the other patients they need to see, or consult with one another about why I am visiting, despite my having said why, despite companions speaking capably for me when I could not speak. The elevated blood pressure at repeated ED visits, for a history of 2 years, was not enough. Kind, straightforward communication is no longer possible in the broader, contemporary context of North America's opioid epidemic. Inside this brown body, there are other things than my pain level to consider: my clothing, my hair, my use of words, and my child's appearance if she was with me. And when they had time to listen, I remembered what they did: one squatted to my eye level to tell me they learned that my condition represents a small percentage of the population (according to the World Health Organization), another encouraged me to find a pain specialist because it would reduce trips to the ED and ease my visits when I did come, a nurse whispered in telling me it was right to come in when an organ shuts down (no matter what a doctor could or could not do about it), and still others who bothered to wave and wish me well with a class, a workout goal, or any detail we'd exchanged when I left, able again to stand on my own two feet. As a patient, I depended on my providers to care for me, to partner with me in care.

The clinical implications for Stang et al.'s research [1] is the "importance of encouraging the use of a validated pain scale and conducting and documenting pain reassessments. It is imperative that pain not only be measured with a valid, objective tool but also be frequently reassessed to optimize pain management." For brown-bodied persons, pain scales have to be taken into account not only in terms of the scale itself, or even in the present event of a visit to the ED. For working bodies, embedded in families and also in environments that are unsympathetic to the realities of daily existence in a racially oppressive society, pain scales must more accurately account for functions, stamina, and time data points for activity. North American medicine's current focus on functionality, in terms of opioid prescriptions, is a legitimate physiological concern; but in balance, the sustenance of pain under persistent conditions of duress is significant and not unrelated to practices and conditions that lead to comorbidities associated with COVID-19 vulnerability to death.

Clinical implications also include ED crowding, which is most common in urban settings with high concentrations of low-income, racial minorities—many of whom are either uninsured or insured by ACA. While it seems unlikely that a busy ED nurse would be unable to collect this information without a more lengthy conversation, it is possible to add these questions to another role of checking in with the patient (during their visit to the ED) or as immediate follow-up by phone in the following day. According to Stang et al. "it is clear that awareness and documentation of pain and its management are, at best, suboptimal":

> …the development of patient-centred outcome indicators and *work linking process measures to these patient outcomes* [my emphasis] would help to clarify the degree to which our current analgesia practices impact the patient.

A key finding in the Stang et al. research is that 91% (ninety-one percent) of the identified indicators were specific to presenting pain only, and a lack of measures reflecting patient-focused outcomes. "The relative lack of indicators for procedural pain highlights a significant gap in measurement and a potential missed opportunity for quality improvement."

Critiques of narrative medicine include whether or not it can be feasibly implemented, and if so, in what role and how to compile the information and share it widely and ethically. Narrative medicine is also criticized for being unreliable as a retrospective methodology for compiling information on individual health [19]: "Retrospective data cannot account for patient preference, pain perception, and appropriate medical justifications for avoiding analgesia." But qualitative methods in health practice and research are much needed for a greater depth of understanding into the processes by which providers and patients properly identify, treat, and manage care. In particular, where patient demographics are incongruous with that of providers, greater training for listening, empathy, and follow-up care are needed for the effective management of pain, especially in brown-bodied patients for whom practices are lacking as indicated in by research evidence.

Conclusion

This "story" is a journey of pain identification, treatment, and management, but it is also a story about the practice of care, the institutions that manage health, and the providers who make a difference in that care. If healthcare providers are to advance the quality of care for individuals in an already complex system, narratives must become a greater part of the innovation that shapes biomedical and social transformations fittingly for those who hold an already complicated relationship with healthcare providers. In this writing, I offer mine as a starting point for medical students and professionals thinking through the problem of brown-bodied pain in North American society.

References

1. Stang, A. S., Hartling, L., Fera, C., Johnson, D., & Ali, S. (2014). Quality indicators for the assessment and management of pain in the emergency department: A systematic review. *Pain Research & Management, 19*(6), e179–e190.
2. O'Mahony, S. (2013). Against narrative medicine. *Perspectives in Biology and Medicine, 56*(4), 611–619.
3. Centers for Disease Control and Prevention (CDC). CDC 24/7: Saving Lives and Protecting People. "Opioid Overdose". 2017. https://www.cdc.gov/drugoverdose/index.html. Accessed 03 Jan 2018.
4. Kalitzkus, V., & Matthiessen, P. F. (2009). Narrative-based medicine: Potential, pitfalls, and practice. *The Permanente Journal, 13*(1), 80–86.
5. Fields, K., & Fields, Barbara Jeanne. (2012). Racecraft: The soul of inequality in American life. In Karen E. Fields & Barbara J. Fields (eds.), London; New York: Verso.

6. Tervalon, M., & Murray-García, J. (1998). Cultural humility versus cultural competence: A critical distinction in defining physician training outcomes in multicultural education. *Journal of Health Care for the Poor and Underserved, 9*(2), 117–125.

7. Gravlee, C. (2009). How race becomes biology: Embodiment of social inequality. *American Journal of Physical Anthropology, 139*(1), 47–57.

8. Charon, R. (2006). Narrative medicine : honoring the stories of illness. Oxford University Press.

9. Washington, H. (2006). Medical apartheid : the dark history of medical experimentation on Black Americans from colonial times to the present. Doubleday.

10. Centers for Disease Control and Prevention (CDC). CDC 24/7: Saving lives and protecting people. "Presidential Apology". 1997. https://www.cdc.gov/tuskegee/clintonp.html. Accessed 03 Jan 2018.

11. Skloot, R. (2010). The immortal life of Henrietta lacks. In Rebecca Skloot (ed.), New York: Crown.

12. Wailoo, K. (2014). *Dying in the city of the blues: Sickle cell anemia and the politics of race and health.* University of North Carolina Press.

13. Singhal, A., Tien, Y. Y., & Hsia, R. Y. (2016). Racial-ethnic disparities in opioid prescriptions at emergency department visits for conditions commonly associated with prescription drug abuse. *PLoS ONE, 11*(8), e0159224. https://doi.org/10.1371/journal.pone.0159224

14. Pouget, E. R., Fong, C., & Rosenblum, A. (2018). Racial/ethnic differences in prevalence trends for heroin use and non-medical use of prescription opioids among entrants to opioid treatment programs, 2005–2016. *Substance Use & Misuse, 53*(2), 290–300.

15. Clarke, A. E., et al. (2010). Biomedicalization technoscience, health, and illness in the U.S. In Adele E. Clarke (ed.) (*E-Duke books scholarly collection*). Durham, NC: Duke University Press.

16. U.S. Department of Health and Human Services. Office of minority health. Profile: Black/ African Americans. https://minorityhealth.hhs.gov/omh/browse.aspx?lvl=3&lvlid=61. Accessed 03 Jan 2018.

17. Hiromi, T., Hawks, C., Herrara-Nicol, S., Adams, R., Johnson, B., Sobotka, S., and Jenkins, A. 2020. "Modification of the Castellvi Classification System with a Guide Towards Treatment Decision Making for Bertolotti's Syndrome," presentation at the AANS Annual Meeting, Boston, MA.

18. Arntfield, S., Dickson, J., & Charon, R. (2013). Narrative medicine as a means of training medical students toward residency competencies. *Patient Education and Counseling, 91*(3), 280–286.

19. Green, C. R. (2011). Being present: The role of narrative medicine in reducing the unequal burden of pain. *Pain, 152*(5), 965–966.

20. Jancuska, J. M., Spivak, J. M., & Bendo, J. A. (2015). A review of symptomatic lumbosacral transitional vertebrae: Bertolotti's syndrome. *International Journal of Spine Surgery, 9*, 42. https://doi.org/10.14444/2042.

Monica D. Griffin, Ph.D. is Director of Engaged Scholarship and the Sharpe Community Scholars Program at William and Mary and an Affiliate Faculty in American Studies. She specializes in community studies, teaching community-based, participatory action research methods, health inequality, and theories of culture, race, and social justice. Monica's research interests include cultural sociology, health inequality (and narrative medicine), and community partnering and action research to study inequality in a variety of organizational settings, including higher education.

Chapter 9
Models of Community Care

Paige Rentz, Michelle Douglas, and Renay Scales

During a 2019 Conference on Communities of Practice in Nashville, Tennessee hosted by Meharry Medical College and supported by Health Resources and Service Administration (HRSA), best practices for community medicine were showcased. Two (2) of these programs are represented in this chapter in an effort to address designs that can be considered for replication as we address cultural issues in healthcare. Data has been collected from interviews with individuals directing these programs in the aftermath of the conference.

An interview with Dr. Katherine Y. Brown, director of communities of practice and dissemination for the National Center on Medical Education, Development and Research at Meharry Medical College in Nashville, Tennessee.

Dr. Katherine Y. Brown describes her day-to-day work at the National Center on Medical Education, Development and Research as a kaleidoscope. Her days range from meetings focused on farm worker care to social media training, from planning and presenting at conferences to finding and recruiting experts in the center's research areas.

"In my role, I have to keep thinking what's next," she said. At its core, that multifaceted role focuses on working with teams invested in informing, reviewing, distilling, and disseminating new findings and learning tools developed from the center's many research projects. But for Brown, the learning has been as much through the center's process as its research products.

P. Rentz (✉)
Center for Leadership and Social Change, Florida State University, Tallahassee, FL, USA
e-mail: prentz@fsu.edu

M. Douglas
Human Resources and EDI, Florida State University, Tallahassee, FL, USA
e-mail: mbdouglas@fsu.edu

R. Scales
University of Kentucky College of Medicine (Formerly), Lexington, KY, USA

© The Author(s), under exclusive license to Springer Nature   155
Switzerland AG 2023
R. Scales, A. T. McCleary-Gaddy (eds.), *Cultural Issues in Healthcare*,
https://doi.org/10.1007/978-3-031-20826-3_9

The Project

The National Center on Medical Education, Development and Research at Meharry Medical College was one of six projects funded by the Health Resources and Services Administration of the US Department of Health and Human Services. Going into the 5-year project, Brown said, the National Center on Medical Education, Development and Research had very specific primary goals:

- to examine and explore the evidence for effective medical education and clinical practice in the treatment of identified vulnerable populations,
- to identify levels of adaptation of evidence-based best practices in primary care training,
- to disseminate best practices through curriculum recommendations, webinars, conferences, and social media.

Now in its 5th year, the NCMEDR has completed research projects on 10 distinct topics, each of which is applicable to all three of the center's identified vulnerable populations: migrant farm workers, members of the LGBTQ community, and people experiencing homelessness.

Communities of Practice

The Model

A community of practice is a model of social learning in which the participants acknowledge that their shared focus on a topic creates learning potential for the group (Wenger). Brown referenced this model in explaining the function of communities of practice in the center's work. Each is built around a domain or the shared interest or passion to which members are committed. This does not mean simply a group of friends or like-minded individuals, Brown emphasized, as members of the COP are committed to its work.

In the aspect of community, members with different backgrounds and experiences build relationships that enable them to learn from each other (Wenger). At the center, the COPs met regularly—sometimes as often as weekly—in an effort to build community and move the process forward.

"It was really important to make sure that the voices were all represented," Brown said. "When you think about a community of practice, it's not just all researchers or academicians, you have to have stakeholders, you have to have people who represent the vulnerable population, you have to have caregivers, students—so there's a very diverse lens."

Diversity was critical not only among the COP members as a whole but also among stakeholders that were members of the vulnerable populations themselves.

Making sure that there was a representation of people of various backgrounds and identities was critical for Brown. She also noted that in some cases, membership in the vulnerable populations overlaps; for example, someone who is part of the LGBTQ community may have experienced homelessness because they were kicked out of their home because of their identity.

"You can't look at it through a single lens because life isn't in a single lens," she said.

The quest to continually diversify the communities of practice led Brown to continually employ her favorite question with members: "This was a great meeting," Brown would say, "but who's missing at the table?" This effort to add new voices and perspectives, she said, "is really how we grew, we evolved, and we defined ourselves."

The final aspect of practice includes the interactions that build over time and help members learn together.

"Everyone has a voice of equal amplification at the table," Brown said, "so everyone is a practitioner regardless of what your degree says you are; you have a vested interest in this group."

The Center has a staff of about 15 people, but the COP model ensures much more input. Each COP has a faculty consultant with expertise in the subject area, and the center has national partnerships with three large nonprofit institutions—The Migrant Clinician's Network, National Healthcare for the Homeless Council, and the Fenway Institute's National LGBTQIA+ Health Education Center—and a number of partnerships with local and regional organizations. In addition, each community of practice has about 30 members, anywhere from 60 to 100 members gather at the annual COP conference where that year's research is presented, and nearly 200 people have served in the COPs since the project began.

The Process

While research is the core of the project, according to Brown, the findings are just the first piece of the puzzle. The overarching process hinges on successfully translating researchers' results and getting recommendations to stakeholders in ways they will actually consume and integrate the information.

"I think that honestly to exclude the beauty of the COP really takes away from the strategic and systematic process that went into the 5-year project," Brown said.

Brown serves a dual role in this process, both as the convener of the communities of practice and as the Center's director with responsibility for disseminating the information that ultimately develops from their work. Once the research teams convene and produce their findings, Brown, wearing her COP director hat, would join the process and bring together the communities for members' feedback on how the research can be utilized. In other words, the examination of research findings goes beyond the research team's evaluation to even more critically determine how the group stakeholders feel about the efficacy of the application. Brown comments on the excitement of these exchanges and the uniqueness of this approach.

Making use of the research, the communities of practice work together to give feedback and generate ideas for the next steps, and then Brown, now working in her capacity as director of dissemination, would help get this information out to a wide range of audiences.

"I was looking at academic, professional, clinical, consumers—how do we translate this information in terms of what we're learning?" Brown said. The answer turned out to be an array of methods, with social media becoming Brown's favorite means of spreading the message.

Social Recruitment

As Brown continually returned to the question of "Who's missing?" throughout her work with the COPs, she was able to find some answers through social media. Researching and using popular hashtags for the topics of the center's research led Brown to discover new voices—content experts and other stakeholders—who she could message through the platforms to recruit them for a COP or other help in the project. "That's the power of social media," she said.

Brown even reached out to Etienne Wenger, the prominent social learning theorist known for his work related to communities of practice, for his expert feedback on the center's implementation of the model. This led to Wenger conducting a webinar for the center and appearances at the annual COP conference and a meeting of the HRSA grantees, she said.

"That was an exciting aspect of 'How do we utilize technology and social media, and what does that mean?'" Brown said. "We research people, we research their concepts, but how often do we reach out to them and say, 'I want to know I am doing this work the right way, the way that you envisioned it,' and to get that feedback is absolutely priceless."

Dissemination

Perhaps the most critical aspect of the center's dissemination strategy was that the communities of practice were really guiding the process. Listening, building rapport, and establishing trust were critical components of the process that intersected every topic, Brown said. From there, it was about the art of communication. Those aspects intersected as she sought innovative ways to make sure information got to each of the center's audiences, especially in instances when "a selfie of you getting something done [would be] more powerful than me putting out a 20-page PDF that nobody's ever going to read," she said.

Consistent Messaging and Building Trust

In a process with so many stakeholders, consistent messaging was critical. Brown developed training for center faculty and other stakeholders on how to use social media specifically in ways to spread messages related to their research topics and identified vulnerable populations for a wide array of audiences. Throughout the process, Brown continued her own development as well, receiving bronze, silver, and gold fellowship awards from completing the Mayo Clinic Social Media Network for her social media work with the National Center and completing Mayo's social media residency in year three of the center's project. She has gone on to serve as a peer leader for the residency, a webinar and conference presenter, and a member of the external advisory board for the program.

An important realization for Brown during her work with the communities of practice was getting to the root of a very basic question: Why should people trust you? It was important to the center for members of vulnerable populations to be able to see themselves reflected in various ways in the center's work and messaging. Using social media, Brown researched health holidays and various national recognition days related to each of the groups, such as Transgender Day of Visibility, and included those in the center's social media plans, both to share content and amplify the voices of those groups.

Many COP members expressed frustration at the number of people who wanted them to sign research waivers for their stories in exchange for groceries or supplies that were not useful in their circumstances, Brown said. So continually building trust through authentic interactions and messaging was important; they had to "walk the walk" as much as they "talked the talk" when it came to listening to people they serve. The center also took other simple but critical steps such as using person-first language and researching imagery, colors, and other culturally appropriate nuance for representation in various media.

"If they couldn't look and see themselves in the social media, and they couldn't see where we were using their stories, if they couldn't come to that conference and see themselves reflected, it was a problem," Brown said.

Establishing trust with COP members paved the way for more powerful storytelling, Brown said. One outcome of the process was the creation of "clinical vignettes"—recorded conversations with COP members about their personal experiences in healthcare settings, which are used as part of facilitated discussions, often at national conferences.

The COP members often recount stories that range from frustrating to traumatic, providing insight into how their interactions with healthcare professionals impacted them. And in the conference setting, Brown encourages participants to develop a "simple message that inspires," finding their own personal call to action from the video, whether it is sharing information on social media or aiming at broader structural change.

"Providers, medical students, social workers, everyone who saw the vignettes talked about how impactful it was," Brown said. And as the clinical vignettes continue to be used in these ways, Brown continues to ask what the center can learn from this process and apply it to transforming medical education. The vignettes will soon be used as a training tool for students at Meharry, Brown said, and the center is currently working to create a portal so that colleagues nationwide will be able to use the center's curriculum modules.

"Traditional" Outlets

That the center was constantly searching for new and innovative ways to disseminate information did not slow the output for more traditional research outlets. Over the 5 years that the national center has been in operation, no fewer than 14 peer-reviewed academic publications have emerged from the research its members have undertaken. Topics of these publications have ranged from screening for violent tendencies in adolescents to the use of implicit bias training to prepare medical students to address the needs of vulnerable patient populations, from publications examining a variety of specific health disparities among vulnerable populations to a framework for primary care training that promotes health equity.

Center staff and researchers have also presented their work at conferences—including several instances at the Health Disparities Conference hosted by Xavier University of Louisiana, as well as those hosted by the American Public Health Association, Association of American Medical Colleges, and Research Centers in Minority Institutions—and hosted dozens of webinars related to their work, reaching more than 630 participants [1]. The center's website, ncmedr.org, is a hub of information, hosting summaries of research projects, literature reviews, policy briefs, and other resources. Through May 2021, more than 11,000 users had visited the center's website more than 865,800 times and viewed nearly 1.49 million pages on the site, according to the site's public user data.

Although social media has become Brown's favored means of dissemination, she is quick to note the importance of meeting various segments of their audience where they are. The center was able to create a cable TV show that aired through Comcast and ATT Uverse and reached an estimated 161,000 households, many in the rural reaches of Middle Tennessee.

Brown said the COPs have helped her think critically about how to disseminate information across specific barriers. For some members of the vulnerable groups, access to social media or other digital platforms may not be consistent because of their living or working environments. In those cases, examining the use of physical media spaces such as billboards or benches becomes more important. "Do I put educational flyers in the food boxes that the local food pantry gives out?" Brown asked.

Getting these messages out in holistic ways that reach everyone, according to Brown, requires thinking outside of (and, perhaps occasionally, right into) the box. "That to me, out of all of the projects, was the 'aha moment' of the community of practice," she said.

Working on this project with the communities of practice has been life-changing for Brown. She has grown as a person during the experience, she said, and has learned so much from the members.

"You don't have to have a certain degree to have a voice," she said, "and I really hope people get that from this process."

Community Medicine Model for the Hispanic/ LatinX Community

As we further consider underserved communities in medicine and healthcare overall, it is important to recognize models that address the needs of one of the largest growing populations in the United States. The Latino/a, Hispanic population in the US National Institutes of Health shows a doubling of the Hispanic population in the US between the census of 1980 and 2000, currently reported over 12%. One community medicine design recognized at the National Conference on Communities of Practice is a design developed by a pediatric physician in Kentucky.

Dr. Janeth Ceballos Osario MD., FAAP, Associate Professor in Pediatrics at the University of Kentucky College of Medicine (UK-COM), was motivated to create Clinica Amiga due to the lack of services specifically for the Hispanic population in the greater Lexington area. Although some services were already provided by using an interpreter in many cases, there was a gap in those to address even more specific needs of the community. The Hispanic population in Fayette County had doubled over the last 15 years, from 3.2% in 2000 to 6.9% in 2015; there are 7661 Hispanic children, according to the US census. This population has historically been underserved, in spite of being mostly covered by Medicaid, and is disproportionately vulnerable to poverty and to adverse developmental, behavioral, and physical health outcomes. In Kentucky, 42% of Hispanics are below the federal poverty level compared to 20% of the general population.

In 2019 Dr. Ceballos created Clinica Amiga, a pediatric medical home for Hispanic/Latinx families in Fayette County, Kentucky which includes not only General Pediatric primary care but also a parent support group in Spanish for Hispanic families with children with special healthcare needs called Un Abrazo Amigo. A health education podcast in Spanish was added to the program and additional outreach activities in the community for health education purposes.

Regarding primary care, the program has made possible the establishment of continuity of care for many Hispanic families who feel more comfortable getting their primary care in Spanish or by a Bilingual provider and staff including Ceballos herself.

The parent support group, Un Abrazo Amigo, has 46 families enrolled with 49 children with special needs. Through the group, parents are provided with monthly healthcare-related educational sessions and a connection with social and community resources helping them to meet other needs of the participating families. Through a monthly health education podcast in Spanish, the program has addressed over 22 different topics available for the local community to hear live every month or at their leisure via the clinic's website. Specific data is collected to be further streamlined, loaded, and tracked in a system whose design is in progress.

Primary care services are provided in a teaching clinic of General Pediatrics at UK-COM. Staff and providers are part of UK Healthcare. The parent support group however is supported by a collaboration between the University of Kentucky, a state grant from the Commission for Children with Special Healthcare Needs and Fayette County Public Schools. The health education podcast is supported by the collaboration between the University of Kentucky and RadioLex, a community radio station.

Potential Breakouts, if Needed

Breakout Box: Methods of Dissemination
- Cable TV show
- Social media

  - Twitter
  - Instagram
  - Facebook
  - YouTube

- Annual Conference
- Presentations
- Policy briefs
- Journal articles
- Webinars

Breakout Box: Research Topics
Year 1:
Implicit Physician Bias
Pre-Exposure Prophylaxis (PrEP)
Year 2:
Interpersonal Violence across the Life Course
Adverse Childhood Experiences

Year 3:
Opioid Misuse
Sexual Violence
Year 4:
Affirming Care
Immunization Disparities
Year 5:
Mental Health
Telehealth

Appendix: Brochure on Program

https://ukhealthcare.uky.edu/kentucky-childrens-hospital/services/primary-care-pediatrics/clinica-amiga

    https://ukhealthcare.uky.edu/wellness-community/blog/clinica-amiga-language-barriers-come-down-hispanic-pediatric-patients

Reference

1. Dissemination. National Center for Medical Education Development and Research. n.d. [cited 2021 May 30]. Available from: https://ncmedr.org/interactive-mapping-2/dissemination/

Paige Rentz,   M.S. is a communications professional at Florida State University's Center for Leadership and Social Change. She also co-leads the university's National Coalition Building Institute affiliate team, TEDxFSU program, and Queer & Trans Employee Network. She is a graduate of Chipola College, Sarah Lawrence College, and the Columbia University Graduate School of Journalism.

Michelle Douglas,   M.S. serves as the Director of the Florida State University's (FSU) Equity, Diversity, and Inclusion (EDI) office. Her office has oversight and responsibility for institutional Equal Opportunity and Compliance (EOC); Equity, Diversity, and Inclusion (EDI), and the Ombuds Program. She is a career HR and diversity professional and co-leads the FSU National Coalition Building Affiliate. She earned a bachelor's degree in History and African American Studies as a student-athlete at the University of Minnesota—Twin Cities, as well as a master's degree in History from Florida State University.

Chapter 10
Final Thoughts

Asia T. McCleary-Gaddy

As a result of the current shift in the United States population demographics, coupled with the ongoing inequities in health care and health outcomes, diversity has been increasingly recognized as a core value in health care through leading organizations such as the Institute of Medicine (2010) and the National League for Nursing (2013). Understanding and eliminating health inequities requires a close examination of our past practice and future focus in healthcare practice research [1]. The method in which we examine the social and structural determinants of health that contribute to inequities requires a study of the environment, context, and *culture* of those experiencing these disparities [1].

One approach to understanding the role of culture in health equity is to employ a pedagogy of cultural humility. Tervalon and Murray-Garcia [2] coined the term "cultural humility" to describe a lifelong process of self-reflection and self-critique whereby the individual not only learns about another's culture, but starts with an examination of her/his own beliefs and cultural identities. This critical consciousness is more than just self-awareness, but requires one to step back to understand one's own assumptions, biases, and values [3]. Using introspection, individuals look at their own background and social environment and how it has shaped their experience. This process recognizes the dynamic nature of culture since cultural influences change over time and vary depending on location. Therefore, cultural humility cannot be reduced to a single curriculum or workshop. Rather it is viewed as an ongoing process.

Similar to how diversity necessitates cultural humility in our patient care, so does cultural humility then engender *advocacy* in patient care and research. According to Tervalon and Murray-Garcia [2] cultural humility also "redresses the power

A. T. McCleary-Gaddy (✉)
Diversity and Inclusion, McGovern Medical School at the University of Texas Health Science Center, Houston, TX, USA
e-mail: Asia.T.McClearyGaddy@uth.tmc.edu

© The Author(s), under exclusive license to Springer Nature Switzerland AG 2023
R. Scales, A. T. McCleary-Gaddy (eds.), *Cultural Issues in Healthcare*,
https://doi.org/10.1007/978-3-031-20826-3_10

imbalances in the physician-patient dynamic, and develops mutually beneficial and non-paternalistic partnerships with communities on behalf of individuals and defined populations." In other words, in order to truly embody cultural humility, there must be widespread acceptance of marginalized patient and community advocacy as a professional obligation. For example, the *American Nursing Association* explicitly states that advocacy is a pillar of nursing [4]. Nurses instinctively advocate for their patients, in their workplaces, and in their communities; but legislative and political advocacy is no less important to advancing the profession and patient care.

In 2001, the *Declaration of Professional Responsibility*, the American Medical Association (AMA) explicitly endorsed that physicians must "advocate for the social, economic, educational, and political changes that ameliorate suffering and contribute to human well-being." In 2002, related to the AMA endorsement, *the American Board of Internal Medicine*, in its charter on medical professionalism, called for a "commitment to the promotion of public health and preventive medicine, as well as public advocacy on the part of each physician [5]. And in 2012, the *International Council of Nurses—Code of Ethics* emphasized the need for nurses to respect the rights, values, customs, and beliefs of individuals and families, and to advocate for equity and social justice in resource allocation and in access to health care [6].

Moreover, as we are still experiencing the two ongoing pandemics of 2020 including COVID-19 and anti-Black and anti-Asian racism in America, organizations have also become more specific in identifying the structural determinants of health and advocating for their elimination within the health professions [6, 7]. In 2020, as an example of these two convening dynamics, the *American Public Health Association* declared that "Racism is a public health and the *Association of American Medical Colleges* [8] stated, "Our country must unite to combat and dismantle racism and discrimination in all its forms and denounce race-related violence, including police brutality. Enough is enough. Racism is antithetical to the oaths and moral responsibilities we accepted as health professionals who have dedicated our lives to advancing the health of all, especially those who live in vulnerable communities."

Earnest et al. [9] coined the term "physician advocacy" to describe an action by a physician to promote those social, economic, educational, and political changes that ameliorate the suffering and threats to human health and well-being that he or she identifies through his or her professional work and expertise. Funk, Hefferon, Kennedy, and Johnson [10] found that public trust of physicians is very high compared to medical researchers since doctors are perceived as a credible source of information. Given this social standing, physicians have higher access to policymakers, to local and national leaders, and to citizens [11]. Therefore, they possess a great deal of leverage in influencing public processes and priorities.

Moreover, past research conducted by Choi [12] suggests that nurses are also uniquely positioned to serve as public advocates for health. Nurses are colloquially referred to as "gatekeepers"for patients since they provide 24-hour continuity of care and close surveillance. As a result, there is evidence that advocacy is inherent to nursing [13] and that a nurse may be in the best position to advocate for the interests and well-being of patients and their communities [15].

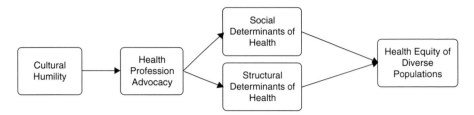

Fig. 10.1 The connection of culture to health equity

Missed Opportunities: A Call to Action

In its landmark report *Closing the Gap in a Generation: Health Equity Through Action on the Social Determinants of Health*, the Commission on Social Determinants of Health (SDOH) described social justice as "a matter of life and death" and that addressing inequities of SDOH is part of social justice [14]. As the author explains in Fig. 10.1, all elements of diversity, culture, and determinants of health are connected in a process toward one goal of health equity. But we cannot continue to miss the opportunities for advancement.

Advocacy in Theory but not Practice

Campbell et al. [16] have noted a discrepancy exists between the professional values health professionals endorse and the behaviors they demonstrate. Specifically, physicians *endorse* the idea of civic engagement as a professional responsibility however are less likely to *engage* in the aforementioned activities. Moreover, research suggests that on the most basic measure of civic involvement, that is, voting, doctors vote less often than other professions or public at large [17]. Physicians and health professionals alike must start changing their behavior to enact the power in advocacy that they hold.

Fragmented vs. Holistic Curriculum

Despite a growing understanding of the importance of SDOH, the inclusion of this material into standard training curricula remains sporadic, and when it is included, it is often considered optional [18]. Tiwari and Palatta [19] suggest that health workforce education and training might consider an interprofessional approach to integrating SDOH into health education and begin shifting away from a biomedical-centric training model to one that incorporates a more holistic approach to addressing the fundamental needs of their patients [20].

Faculty Development vs. a Faculty Tax

In addition to the resources provided by health professions national organizations, academic health institutions can invest in their faculty members' knowledge of SDOH by providing institution-specific professional development opportunities. In reality, much of the teaching load on the SDOH falls on the responsibility of minority faculty of color. In the academic literature, this is referred to as the minority tax; the tax of extra responsibilities placed on minority faculty in the name of efforts to achieve diversity [21]. Health professional school personnel may perform a cultural audit of their learning environments to examine the need for cultural change in the curriculum and the institutional environment [22]. Buy-in from senior leadership is essential in creating a positive environment for change. All faculty members must be involved in understanding the goals associated with the teaching of SDOH concepts via an integrated approach. Utilizing early adopters and faculty champions as role models and mentors for other faculty members has proven to be a successful model.

Research Community Engagement

Americans express less optimism about how often they can count on medical scientists to provide fair and accurate information and to show concern for the public's or patients' interests [10]. Overall, Americans rate researchers more negatively than practitioners when it comes to the trustworthiness of their information. Some have suggested that lingering concerns among Black Americans and other minority communities may be due to the history of mistreatment including the Tuskegee study, and the Puerto Rico birth control study. In health research, cultural stereotypes and assumptions derived from notions of difference find their way into explanations of study findings [23]. Researchers often explain their findings and base their conclusions on making assumptions about cultural groups.

The power imbalance between the researcher and participant must be recognized and minimized in the research process [24]. Cultural humility calls on individuals to be flexible and humble enough to let go of the false sense of security that stereotyping brings and to explore the cultural dimensions of the experiences of each person.

Conclusion

The subsection above is a sample of some of the missed opportunities experienced across health professions and should not be viewed as exhaustive. Collectively, the authors of "Emerging Cultural Issues in Healthcare" are calling on you, the reader, to develop a cultural consciousness for marginalized communities and to be an advocate, or more appropriately—a leader, for health equity and organizational change for our more diverse present and future. While we have explored a number of emerging issues relate to cultural issues in health care, we purport that there is much more work to do to uncover or discover more ways to avert our usual practices and bring forth more positive communication and treatment strategies.

References

1. Yeager, K. A., & Bauer-Wu, S. (2013). Cultural humility: Essential foundation for clinical researchers. *Applied Nursing Research, 26*(4), 251–256.
2. Tervalon, M., & Murray-Garcia, J. (1998). Cultural humility versus cultural competence: A critical distinction in defining physician training outcomes in multicultural education. *Journal of Health Care for the Poor and Underserved, 9*(2), 117–125.
3. Kumagai, A. K., & Lypson, M. L. (2009). Beyond cultural competence: Critical consciousness, social justice, and multicultural education. *Academic Medicine, 84*(6), 782–787.
4. ANA. (n.d.). Advocacy. Retrieved 24 Nov 2021, from https://www.nursingworld.org/practice-policy/advocacy/.
5. ABIM Foundation; ACP-ASIM Foundation. (2002). European Federation of Internal Medicine. Medical professionalism in the new millennium: A physician charter. *Annals of Internal Medicine, 136*, 243–246.
6. International Council of Nurses. (2012). *The ICN code of ethics for nurses.* ICN.
7. Racism is a Public Health Crisis. (n.d.). *Racism declarations: Opportunities for action.* Retrieved 24 Nov 2021, from https://www.apha.org/topics-and-issues/health-equity/racism-and-health/racism-declarations.
8. American Medical Association. (2020). *AMA declaration of professional responsibility.* Retrieved 24 Nov 2021, from https://www.ama-assn.org/delivering-care/public-health/ama-declaration-professional-responsibility.
9. Earnest, M. A., Wong, S. L., & Federico, S. G. (2010). Perspective: Physician advocacy: What is it and how do we do it? *Academic Medicine, 85*(1), 63–67.
10. Funk, C., Hefferon, M., Kennedy, B., & Johnson, C. (2019). Trust and mistrust in Americans' views of scientific experts. *Pew Research Center, 2*, 1–96.
11. Gruen, R. L., Campbell, E. G., & Blumenthal, D. (2006). Public roles of US physicians: Community participation, political involvement, and collective advocacy. *Journal of the American Medical Association, 296*(20), 2467–2475.
12. Choi, P. P. (2015). Patient advocacy: The role of the nurse. *Nursing Standard (2014+), 29*(41), 52.
13. Vaartio, H., Leino-Kilpi, H., Salanterä, S., & Suominen, T. (2006). Nursing advocacy: How is it defined by patients and nurses, what does it involve and how is it experienced? *Scandinavian Journal of Caring Sciences, 20*(3), 282–292.
14. Mallik, M. (1997). Advocacy in nursing—A review of the literature. *Journal of Advanced Nursing, 25*(1), 130–138.
15. CSDH (Commission on Social Determinants of Health). (2008). Closing the gap in a generation: Health equity through action on the social determinants of health. In: *Final report of the commission on social determinants of health.* Geneva, Switzerland: World Health Organization. Available at: https://www.who.int/social_determinants/final_report/csdh_final-report_2008.pdf Accessed 04 Feb 2020.
16. Campbell, E. G., Regan, S., Gruen, R. L., et al. (2007). Professionalism in medicine: Results of a national survey of physicians. *Annals of Internal Medicine, 147*, 795–802.
17. Grande, D., Asch, D. A., & Armstrong, K. (2007). Do doctors vote? *Journal of General Internal Medicine, 22*, 585–589.
18. Siegel, J., Coleman, D. L., & James, T. (2018). Integrating social determinants of health into graduate medical education: a call for action. Academic Medicine, 93(2), 159–62.

19. Tiwari, T., & Palatta, A. M. (2019). An adapted framework for incorporating the social determinants of health into predoctoral dental curricula. *Journal of Dental Education, 83*(2), 127–136. https://doi.org/10.21815/JDE.019.015
20. Frenk, J., Chen, L., Bhutta, Z. A., et al. (2010). Health professionals for a new century: Transforming education to strengthen health systems in an interdependent world. *Lancet, 376*(9756), 1923–1958.
21. Mahoney, M. R., Wilson, E., Odom, K. L., Flowers, L., & Adler, S. R. (2008). Minority faculty voices on diversity in academic medicine: Perspectives from one school. *Journal of the Association of American Medical Colleges, 83*(8), 781–786. https://doi.org/10.1097/ACM.0b013e31817ec002
22. Orfaly, R. A., Frances, J. C., Campbell, P., Whittemore, B., Joly, B., & Koh, H. (2005). Train-the-trainer as an educational model in public health preparedness. *Journal of Public Health Management and Practice, 11*(6), S123–S127.
23. Hunt, L. M., & de Voogd, K. B. (2005). Clinical myths of the cultural "other": Implications for Latino patient care. *Academic Medicine, 80*(10), 918–924.
24. Kvale, S., & Brinkmann, S. (2009). *Interviews: Learning the craft of qualitative research interviewing* (2nd ed.). Sage Publications.
25. Heiser, S. (2020). *AAMC statement on police brutality and racism in America and their impact on health.* AAMC. Retrieved 24 Nov 2021, from https://www.aamc.org/news-insights/press-releases/aamc-statement-police-brutality-and-racism-america-and-their-impact-health

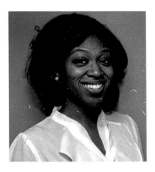

Asia T. McCleary-Gaddy, Ph.D. serves as the Director of Diversity and Inclusion for UTHealth Science Center at Houston and is an Assistant Professor of Psychiatry and Behavioral Sciences for McGovern Medical School. Asia serves the UTHealth community through design and implementation of policies and procedures that support Diversity and Inclusion, recruitment and retention of URM faculty and students, program evaluation and data analysis for students, residents, and faculty members. Dedicated to furthering the empirical research published on diversity and health, she has published in leading journals including Annals of Behavioral Medicine, Journal of Health Psychology, and Equality, Diversity, and Inclusion. Most recently, Dr. McCleary-Gaddy was recognized by the National Diversity Council as a DEI Champion at the Health Equity and Inclusion Conference. Prior to this positon, Dr. McCleary-Gaddy served as the inaugural Director of Diversity and Equity for Hackensack Meridian School of Medicine and helped launch the institutions high school pipeline/pathway programs. Prior to that role, she served as a Data Analyst for the Vermont Department of Health in Burlington, VT where she analyzed data for the Healthy People 2020 initiative. Dr. McCleary-Gaddy earned a PhD in Experimental Social Psychology. She also holds a BA degree in Psychology with a distinction in Research and Creative Works and minor in Poverty, Justice, and Human Capabilities from Rice University. Her research interests include stigmatization, diversity science, and coping mechanisms.

Index